Keto Diet Plan

Clarity, Simply and Easy Guide for Beginners to 21-Day Meal Plan for Weight Loss and Healthy Living with a Keto Lifestyle... with Fat Bombs!

© Copyright 2020 by Meriem Simson - All rights reserved.

The following Book is reproduced below with the goal of providing information that is as accurate and reliable as possible. Regardless, purchasing this Book can be seen as consent to the fact that both the publisher and the author of this book are in no way experts on the topics discussed within and that any recommendations or suggestions that are made herein are for entertainment purposes only. Professionals should be consulted as needed prior to undertaking any of the action endorsed herein.

This declaration is deemed fair and valid by both the American Bar Association and the Committee of Publishers Association and is legally binding throughout the United States.

Furthermore, the transmission, duplication, or reproduction of any of the following work including specific information will be considered an illegal act irrespective of if it is done electronically or in print. This extends to creating a secondary or tertiary copy of the work or a recorded copy and is only allowed with the express written consent from the Publisher. All additional right reserved.

The information in the following pages is broadly considered a truthful and accurate account of facts and as such, any inattention, use, or misuse of the information in question by the reader will render any resulting actions solely under their purview. There are no scenarios in which the publisher or the original author of this work can be in any fashion deemed liable for any hardship or damages that may befall them after undertaking information described herein. Additionally, the information in the following pages is intended only for informational purposes and should thus be thought of as universal. As befitting its nature, it is presented without assurance regarding its prolonged validity or interim quality. Trademarks that are mentioned are done without written consent and can in no way be considered an endorsement from the trademark holder.

Table of Contents

BREAKFAST 16

    Mushroom Omelet 20
    Coconut Pancakes 21
    Pork and Spinach Omelet 23
    Avocado & Sausage 24
    Eggs, Tomato, Bacon Salad 25
    Breakfast Egg Burrito 26
    Bacon, Spinach, and Eggs 28
    Chocolate Almond Smoothie 29
    Avocado Breakfast Bowls 31
    Bacon and Spinach Egg Frittata 32
    Keto Sausage and Egg Sandwich 34
    Keto Philly Cheesesteak Omelet 35
    Chocolate Mint Avocado Shake 37
    Coconut Porridge 41
    Cinnamon Keto Granola 42
    Keto Blueberry Pancakes 43
    Raspberry Avocado Smoothie 45

LUNCH 47

    Zucchini and Avocado Noodles 48
    BLT Lettuce Wraps 49
    Rosemary Chicken w/ Broccoli 50
    Caesar Salad 52
    Turkey Chili 53
    Deli Meat Plate 54
    Kale Beef and Veggie Wrap 55
    Keto Crescent Hot Dogs 57
    Keto Friendly Pizza Rolls 58
    Tuna Salad and Boiled Eggs 60
    20 Minute Meatballs 61
    Avocado Egg Salad 63
    Chicken Cucumber Avocado Salad 64
    Sesame Salad 66
    Keto Tuna Salad 67
    Pesto Chicken Salad 69
    Low-Carb Chicken Nuggets 70
    Taco Casserole 71

Tomato Basil Soup 73
Chocolate Coconut Keto Smoothie 74
Cheesy Bacon Chicken 75

DINNER 76

Steak Stir Fry 77
Grilled Shrimp & Cod Fillet 79
Arugula Caesar Salad 80
Rosemary Pork Roast 81
Broccoli and Bacon with Mushrooms 83
Lettuce Burger 84
Roasted Chicken Leg with Veggies 86
Grilled Chicken with Guacamole 87
Grilled Salmon and Green Beans 89
Mexican Cauliflower Rice 91
Creamy Mushroom Chicken 92
Mushroom Bacon Skillet 94
Stuffed Peppers 95
Cabbage Soup 99
Salmon Patties 100
Mustard Glazed Chicken Thighs 101
Romaine Lettuce Soup 103
Taco Salad Bowl 105
Cauliflower Mac and Cheese 107

What Is the Keto Diet?

The Ketogenic diet, or the Keto diet for short, has become a popular national sensation because of the weight loss results and health benefits it provides! As we explained briefly in the introduction, this diet is low in carbohydrates to push the body into the metabolic state of Ketosis. Ketosis is when the body's liver uses the fat already stored to produce Ketones to use as energy instead of glucose, which is produced from carbohydrates. When a diet consists mainly of carbohydrates, as most diets are, the body's initial process is to produce that into glucose, or sugar molecules, and use that as your energy source. It's the easiest molecule to produce for the body, so it's a quick and "cheap" form of instant energy! Insulin is what sends the glucose throughout the bloodstream. That's why eating too many carbohydrates can cause your blood sugar to spike. There's too much glucose being produced, and more insulin has to be created to assist in moving it. The Ketogenic diet has shown huge reductions in blood sugar and insulin levels for patients who have diabetes or at risk. Along with multiple other health benefits, coupled with weight loss, it's easy to see why this diet has become so popular!

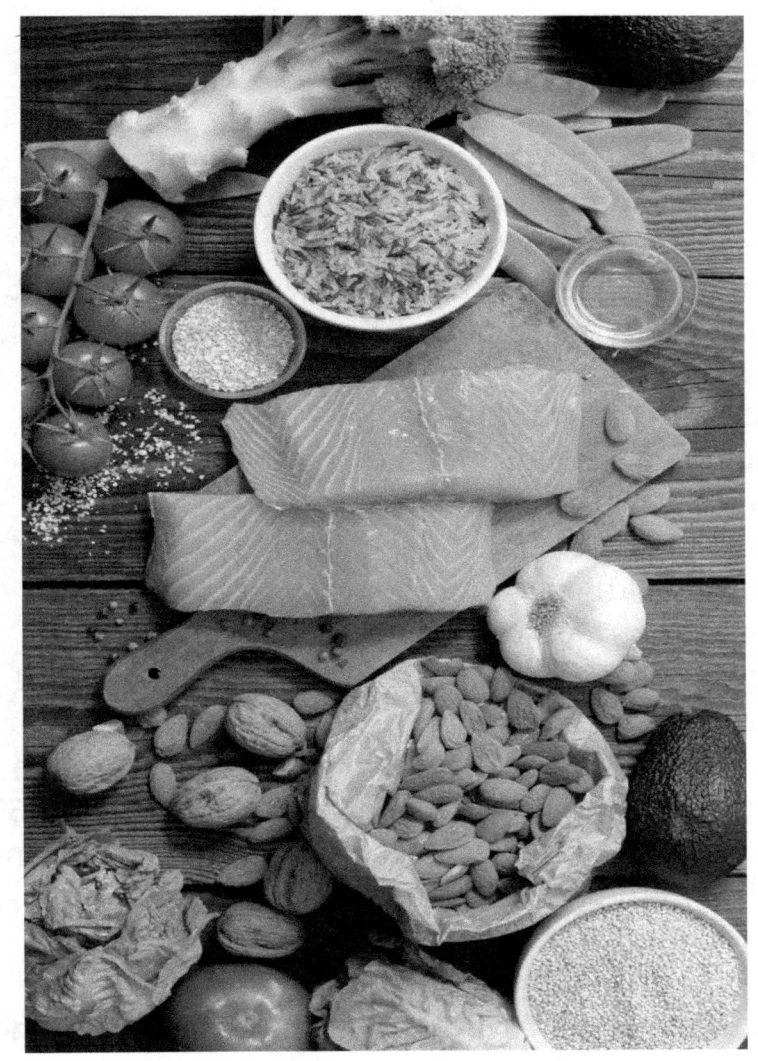

Hence, what are the macro components for a standard Keto diet? For the standard Keto diet that is low-carb, high-fat, and moderate in protein, the breakdown is usually:

75% fat
20% protein
~5% carbs

In most diets, anywhere from 20-30 grams of net carbs is recommended. But keep in mind, the lower you keep your carb intake, the better your overall weight loss results will be. That's why it's important to keep track of your total carbs and macros, especially when you're first starting out and getting familiar with a Keto diet. You want to also ensure you're not overdoing your protein intake and that most of your diet is filled with high-quality fat content.

The diet can be tweaked depending on a person's needs or health concerns. If someone is an athlete and needs extra carbs to complete their workouts, they can follow a more targeted Ketogenic diet that increases their carbs. A high protein Keto diet is similar to the Keto diet but allows for an increase in protein, so it's roughly 60% fat, 35% protein, and 5% carbs. Some people may feel more comfortable doing a cyclical Keto diet where there are certain days they have a higher carb count. It could be 4 days on a strict Keto diet with low carbs and then 2 days with a higher carb count. This can be helpful for people who still need to train themselves to a lower carb count before fully going Keto.

Keep in mind, though, that most of the research has been conducted on the standard Keto diet. Cyclic and targeted Keto diets are more common for athletes or bodybuilders, but they aren't used in most scientific studies. For the purposes of our book, when we mention research and health benefits, we will be referring to the standard Keto diet with a moderate protein count.

There are some critics of the Keto diet who will say that you're pushing your body unnaturally towards a state of Ketosis by decreasing your carb intake so drastically. But that's not it at all! Our bodies are medical marvels that are designed with multiple routes to create energy with the food that we are eating. The only reason the body breaks down carbs into glucose first is that it's so used to that as our energy input. In a normal diet, nearly 65% of the content is carbs! That's what our bodies have gotten used to for creating energy only because carbs are what it's mostly getting. When you change the make-up of your diet, your body will realize there is a shortage of carbs and find an alternative pathway to create energy, which is Ketosis. You already have the energy stored away as fat molecules—it just needs to be used! Our bodies are created to adapt to changes in diet and environmental changes, and stress factors. Think about how our hunters and gatherer ancestors lived. Sometimes famine would occur, and they would have to minimize their diet or even fast so the children and elderly would have food instead. It's just like when you're trying to quit smoking or caffeine. Your body has become adapted and dependent on a certain thing, but you have to be motivated enough to make a change for your health. And when most people see all the health benefits the Keto diet has to offer besides just weight loss, it's a great motivator for them to change their eating habits.

Breakfast

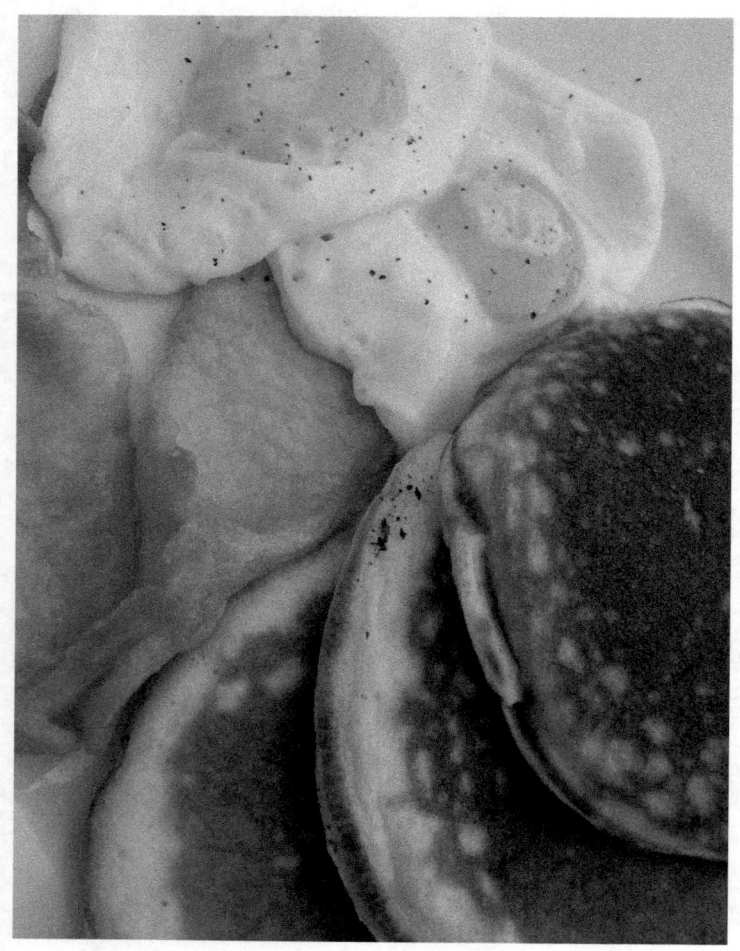

Breakfast Sausage (6 servings; breakfast)
(1 serving: 184 calories, 12.8 grams, 0.28 grams of carbs, 16.08 grams of protein)

Ingredients:
1-pound ground chicken
1-pound ground pork
1 tsp. dried herbs
½ tsp. salt
½ tsp. black pepper
¼ tsp. nutmeg, onion powder, paprika, red chili pepper, and garlic powder

Directions:
In a large bowl, mix together all the ingredients until well-combined.
Portion out 6 hamburger patties. You can eat one as breakfast sausage and keep the others for later in the week or to add on top of a salad for some protein.

Sausage and Eggs (1 serving; breakfast)
(479 calories, 37 grams of fat, 2.5 grams of fiber, 30 grams of protein)

Ingredients:
1 sausage
2 eggs
1 tbsp. olive oil
Salt and pepper to taste
2 asparagus
Directions:
Cut the asparagus in half and cut off the stems.
Boil in some water until tender.
Add ½ tablespoon of olive oil to a small saucepan on medium heat. Then add the asparagus and breakfast sausage and cook on all sides. Transfer to a different plate.
Then add the other half of the olive oil and add the eggs.
Cook covered for a few minutes until the egg whites are completely cooked. Season with salt and pepper.

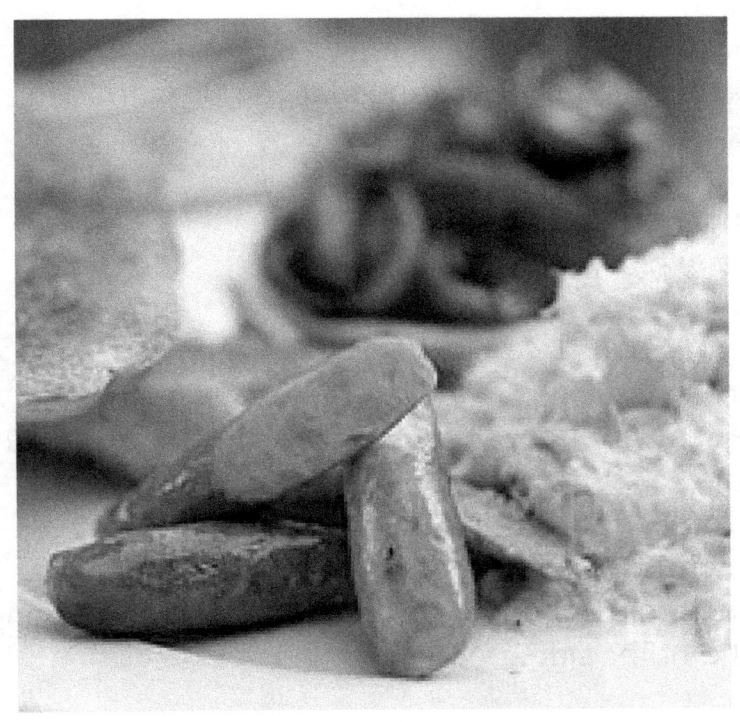

Mushroom Omelet

(1 serving; breakfast)
(510 calories, 40 grams of fat, 28 grams of protein, 6 grams of carbs, 2 grams of fiber)

Ingredients:
1 tbsp. butter for frying
¼ cup shredded cheese, Cheddar, or Mozzarella
3 eggs
4 mushrooms, sliced
Salt and pepper to taste
3 tbsps. white onion, chopped
Directions:
Crack your eggs in a bowl and mix in the salt and pepper.
In a saucepan on low heat, melt the butter and add your egg mixture.
When the edges of the egg begin to crinkle and brown, add the cheese, onion, and mushroom.
Flip the omelet when it has turned golden brown and cook the other side.

Coconut Pancakes

(2 servings total; breakfast)
(1 serving: 578 calories, 50 grams of fat, 20 grams of protein, 3.5 grams of net carbs)

Ingredients:
2 eggs
2 oz. cream cheese, softened
A pinch of salt
A pinch of cinnamon
1 tbsp. almond flour
½–1 tbsp. sweetener substitute

Directions:
Whisk your eggs in a large mixing bowl.
Add in the sweetener, salt, almond flour, cinnamon, and cream cheese and mix until well-combined.
In a skillet on medium heat, add half the pancake batter and let it cook until the edges begin to crinkle and brown. It usually takes about 4–5 minutes, so watch carefully to avoid burning.
Flip to the other side, let it get cooked, then remove from heat. Do this with the rest of the pancake batter to make another pancake. You can add unsweetened coconut flakes or berries as a topping.

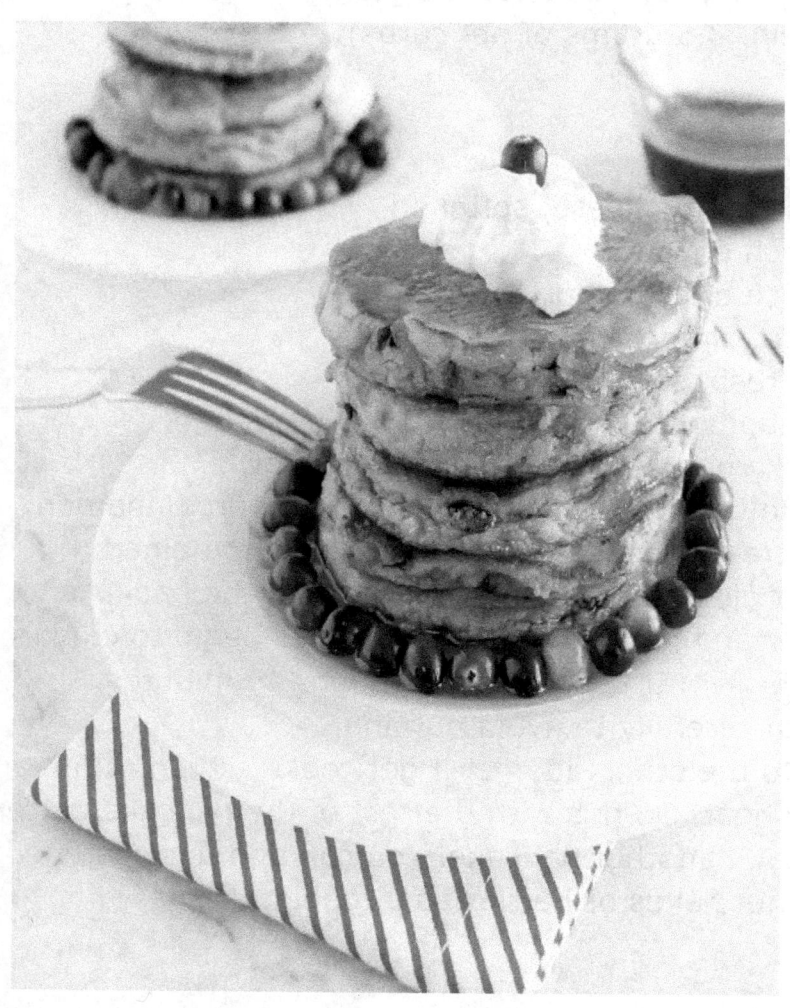

Pork and Spinach Omelet

(1 serving; breakfast)
(425 calories, 4.8 grams of carbs, 0.9 grams of fiber, 27.9 grams of protein)

Ingredients:
1 breakfast sausage
3 eggs
2 tbsps. olive oil
1 garlic clove, minced
¼ red pepper
½ cup spinach leaves
Salt and pepper to taste
Directions:
Crumble the sausage and slice the red pepper finely.
In a large frying pan on medium heat, add the olive oil and cook the sausage until it's golden brown.
Add the garlic, spinach, and pepper to the pan and cook until they become soft.
Crack the eggs in a bowl and season with salt and pepper, and whisk together.
Pour the eggs into the saucepan and let them cook for 4–5 minutes. When the sides of the omelet start to golden brown and crinkle, flip it and cook the other side.

Avocado & Sausage

(1 serving; breakfast)
(524 calories, 11 grams of carbs, 8.3 grams of fiber, 30.79 grams of protein)

Ingredients:
3 pieces sausage
¼ cup spinach
1 tbsp. mayo
Salt and pepper to taste
1–2 asparagus
½ avocado—pitted
1 tsp. olive oil

Directions:
Heat the olive oil in a small pan on medium heat.
Fry the sausages and asparagus until they are cooked and keep in a bowl.
Season the spinach with mayo and salt and pepper and place in your avocado where the pit was.

Eggs, Tomato, Bacon Salad

(1 serving; breakfast)
(524 calories, 40 grams of fat, 1.8 grams of fiber, 36 grams of protein)

Ingredients:
3 slices bacon
2 eggs
1 tsp. olive oil
Salt and pepper to taste
¼ red pepper, sliced
5–8 slices zucchini
3–4 slices tomato
1 basil leaf
1 garlic clove, minced
Directions:
In a saucepan on medium heat, add the olive oil and fry the bacon until golden brown.
Fry the pepper and zucchini until they are soft.
Add the eggs and scramble them until they are cooked. Season everything with salt and pepper.
Remove from heat and keep on a plate.
Add the minced garlic, basil leaf, and tomato.
Add dressing of your choice.

Breakfast Egg Burrito

(1 serving; breakfast)
(522 calories, 44.2 grams of fat, 11 grams of carbs, 21.3 grams of protein)
Ingredients:
2 eggs
1 slice tomato
1 tbsp. mayo
1 lettuce leaf
½ avocado, pitted, peeled, and sliced
2 slices bacon
1 tbsp. olive oil
Directions:
In a frying pan, add half the olive oil. While it's heating, whisk 2 eggs in a bowl.
Pour half the eggs into the pan and let it cook for 4–5 minutes. Repeat on the other side, then the rest of the egg mixture.
Add the rest of the olive oil and fry the bacon until golden brown.
Slice your avocado and tomato and tear up the lettuce.
Add the veggies into each egg omelet, spread the mayo, and you can roll up the egg like a burrito.

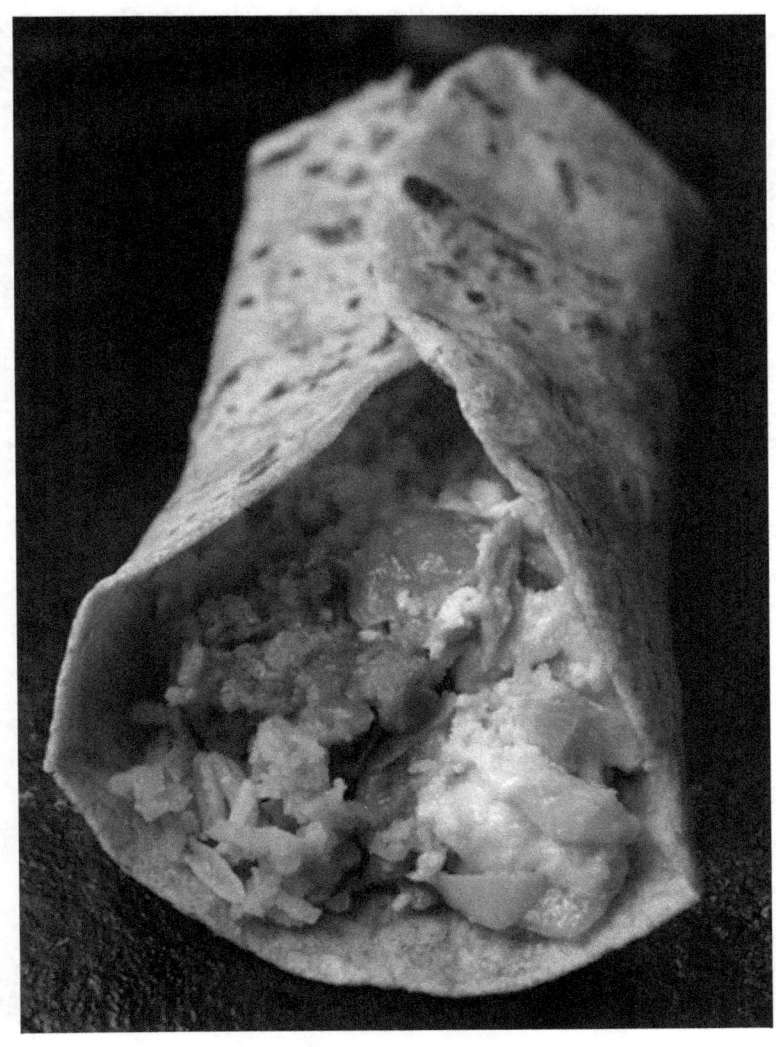

Bacon, Spinach, and Eggs

(1 serving; breakfast)
(366 calories, 2.5 grams of carbs, 0.9 grams of fiber, 27.2 grams of protein)

Ingredients:
Salt and pepper to taste
2 eggs
3 slices bacon
½ cup spinach
1 tbsp. olive oil
Directions:
In a saucepan on medium heat, add the olive oil and fry the bacon until it's crispy.
Chop the spinach roughly and add to the pan where the bacon was. Cook until wilted, then add the eggs over the spinach.
Cover and let them cook for 2–4 minutes until fully cooked.
Sprinkle with salt and pepper and add to the plate with the bacon.

Chocolate Almond Smoothie

(1 serving; breakfast)
(163 calories, 13 grams of total fat, 6.8 grams of carbs, 10 grams of protein, 3 grams of fiber)

Ingredients:
¼ cup cottage cheese
1 ½ tbsp. almond butter or nut butter of your choice
¾ cup water
1 cup unsweetened almond milk
1 tbsp. cocoa powder, unsweetened
3 drops Stevia® liquid
Directions:
Combine all the ingredients in a blender and blend until smooth.

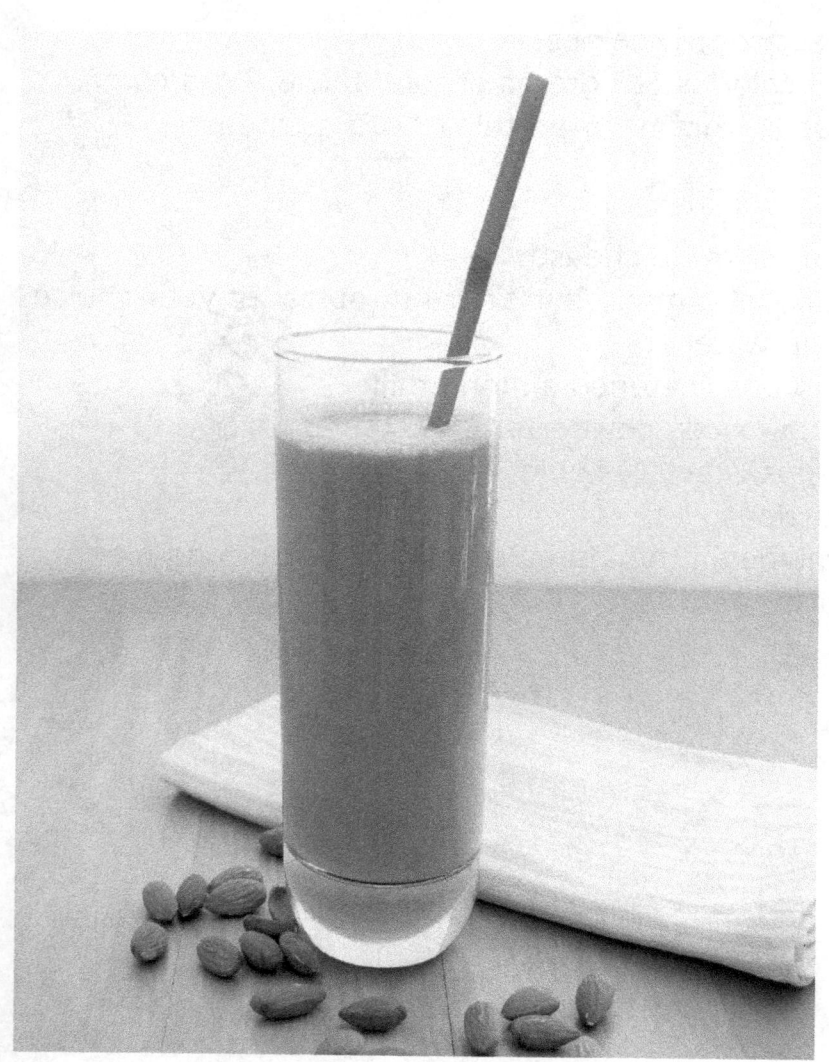

Avocado Breakfast Bowls

(2 servings total; breakfast)
(Per serving: 500 calories, 40 grams of fat, 11 grams of carbs, 8 grams of fiber, 25 grams of protein)

Ingredients:
1 avocado, pitted and halved
3 large eggs
3 slices bacon
A pinch of salt and pepper
1 tbsp. salted butter
Directions:
Scoop out most of the avocado flesh.
In a large saucepan on medium heat, add the butter and let it melt.
While it's melting, crack your eggs into a bowl and season with salt and pepper.
Add bacon to one side of the pan and let it fry until golden brown.
Stir the eggs and bacon together until well-combined. (If one is finished cooking before the other, remove it from the pan and let the other finish cooking.)
Add the mixture into the empty avocado bowls and enjoy.

Bacon and Spinach Egg Frittata

(2 servings; breakfast)
(Per serving: 173 calories, 32 grams of protein, 10 grams of carbs, 32 grams of fat)

Ingredients:
4–5 cherry tomatoes, sliced
1 cups spinach
1 cup green beans
1 tbsp. ghee
4 eggs
4–5 medium-size bacon slices
1 tsp. dried herbs
Directions:
Preheat your oven to 350°F.
In a large saucepan, add the ghee.
Once fragrant, add the bacon and herbs. Cook for 3–4 minutes until golden brown.
Add the vegetables and tomatoes and allow them to soften.
In a bowl, whisk together your eggs and add to the pan. Let them cook until cooked through.
Transfer the pan to the oven and let it bake for another 5–10 minutes until the egg has set.
Slice into 3 portions.

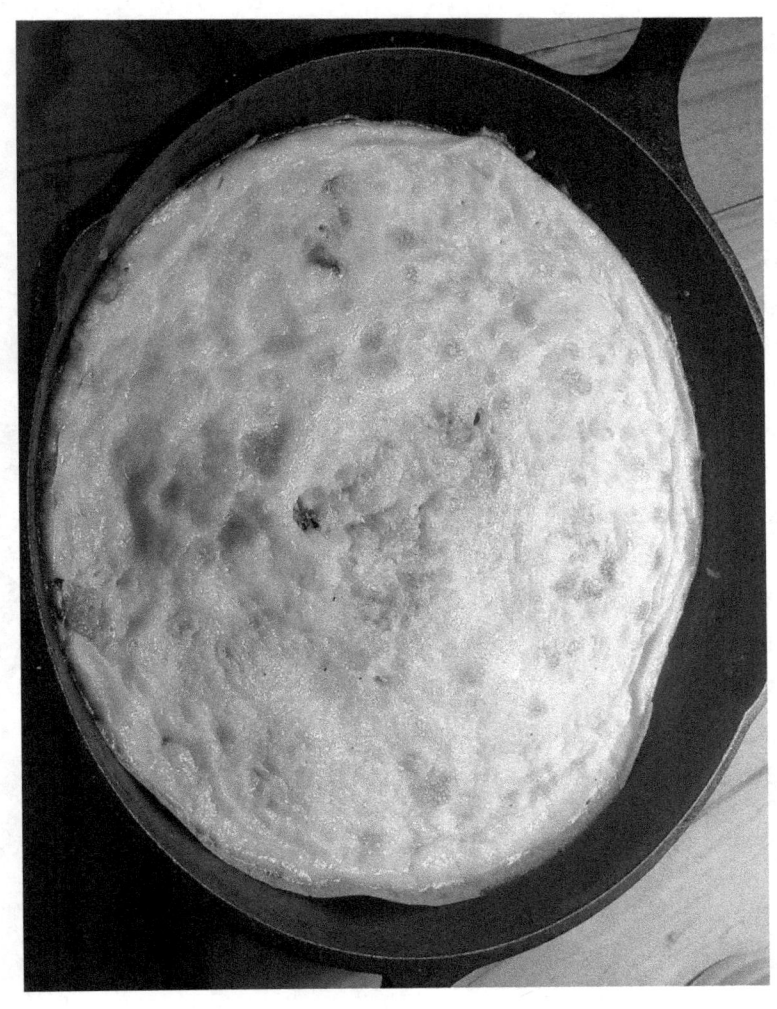

Keto Sausage and Egg Sandwich

(1 serving; breakfast)
(880 calories, 80 grams of fat, 28 grams of protein, 8 grams of carbs, 2 grams of fiber)

Ingredients:
2 slices cheddar cheese
2 sausage patties, cooked
1 tbsp. mayonnaise
2 large eggs
1 tbsp. butter
A few slices tomato
Directions:
Heat the butter in a large skillet over medium heat.
Crack the eggs into the pan and cook for 3–4 minutes, keeping them separate.
Remove from the heat.
Top one egg with half the mayonnaise, and stack your sausage patties, cheese slices, and tomato.
Spread the rest of the mayonnaise on the second cooked egg and add to the top like a burger.

Keto Philly Cheesesteak Omelet

(2 servings total; breakfast)
(Per serving: 418 calories, 32.8 grams of fat, 9 grams of carbs, 28 grams of protein)

Ingredients:
3 oz. provolone, sliced
1 tsp. salt
1 tsp. pepper
¼ pound shaved ribeye
½ green pepper, sliced
½ onion, sliced
2 tbsps. olive oil
4 eggs

Directions:
In a bowl, whisk the eggs and add half the olive oil.
In a skillet over medium heat, pour half the eggs into the pan and cook them through. Cook the other side and then remove from heat.
Repeat with the other half of the egg mixture.
In the same skillet, add the rest of the olive oil and sauté the onion and peppers. Once they become golden brown, transfer to a plate.
Add the meat to the skillet and sauté on medium heat—season with salt and pepper.
Divide the meat into each egg and add the vegetables.

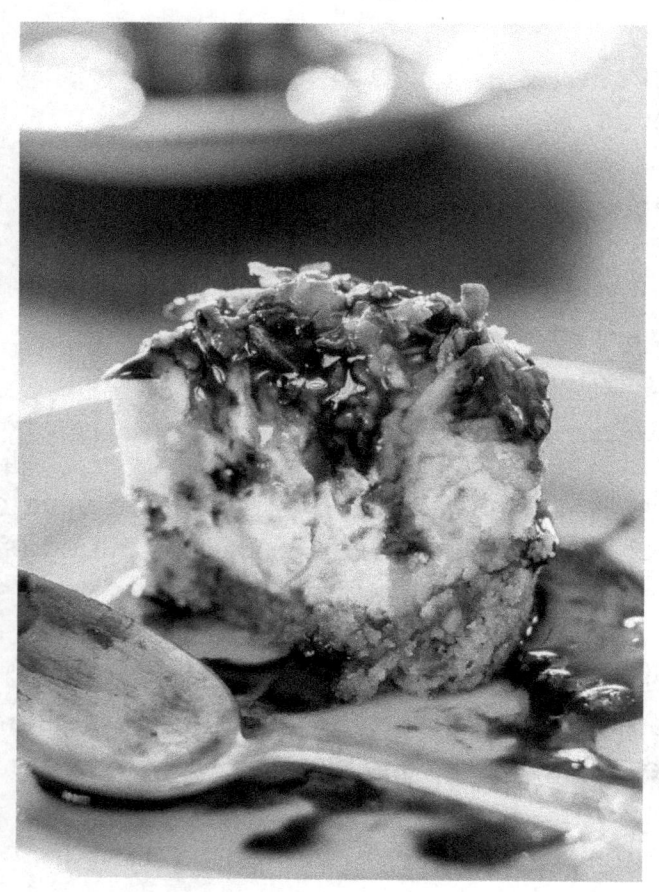

Chocolate Mint Avocado Shake

(1 serving; breakfast)
(528 calories, 24 grams of protein, 10 grams of carbs, 42 grams of fat, 8 grams of fiber)

Ingredients:
A handful ice
½ cup coconut milk
1 cup water
½ avocado—pitted and peeled
4–5 mint leaves
1 tbsp. nut butter
2 tbsps. cacao powder, unsweetened
1 scoop protein powder

Directions:
Add all the ingredients to a blender and blend until smooth.

Avocado, Bacon, and Egg (2 servings total; breakfast)
(Per serving: 128 calories, 9 grams of fat, 8 grams of protein)

Ingredients:
1 medium avocado, pitted and halved
2 eggs
1 tbsp. mozzarella or cheddar cheese
A pinch of salt and pepper
1 piece bacon, cooked and crumbled
Directions:
Preheat your oven to 425°F.
With a tablespoon, scoop out the avocado.
Crack the egg into the avocado and sprinkle with cheese, salt, and pepper, and top with the cooked bacon.
Place on a parchment-lined baking sheet and bake for 14–16 minutes.

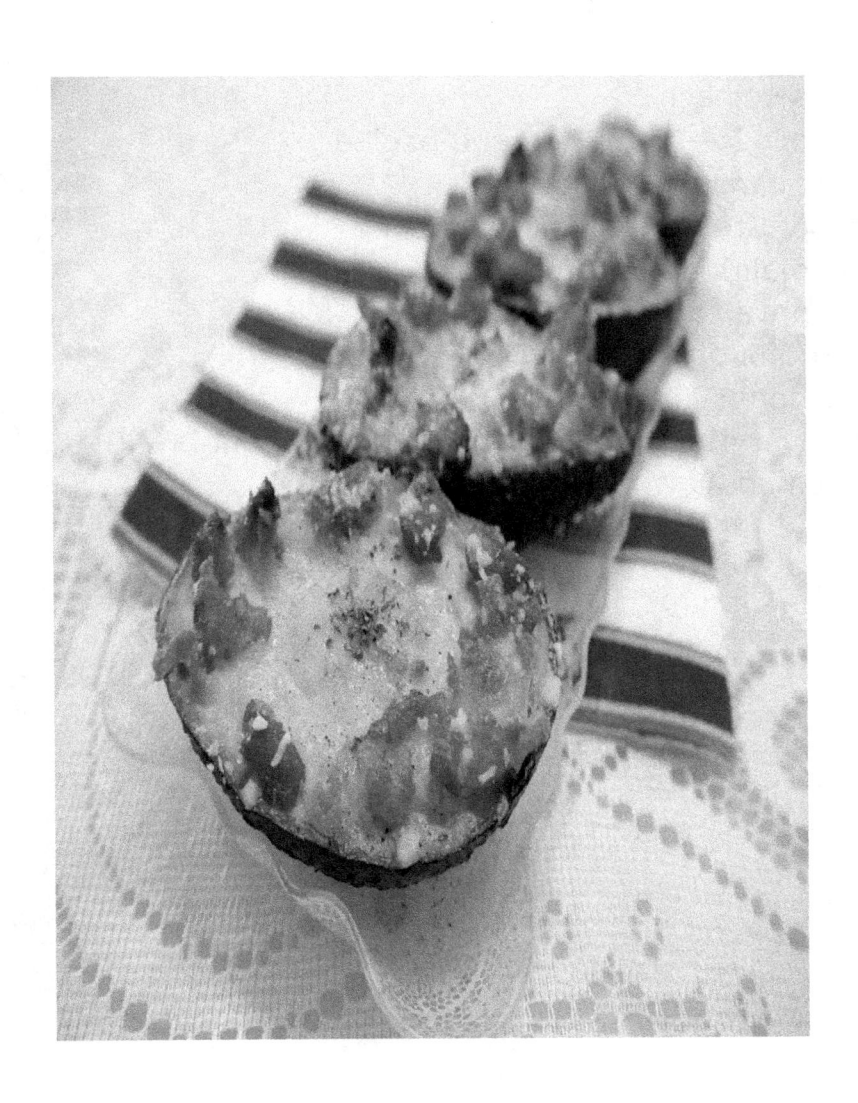

Keto Green Smoothie (1 serving; breakfast)
(263 calories, 23 grams of fat, 10 grams of fiber, 14 grams of carbs, 4.9 grams of protein)

Ingredients:
½ cup spinach
½ avocado—tbsppitted and peeled
1 tsp. vanilla extract
1 tbsp. Stevia® sugar sweetener
½ cup almond milk
½ cup water
A handful of ice
Directions:
Add everything to a blender and blend until well-combined.

Coconut Porridge

(1 serving; breakfast)
(432 calories, 37 grams of fat, 13 grams of carbs, 12 grams of protein)

Ingredients:
1 egg
2 tsp. butter
1 tbsp. Stevia® sugar sweetener
1 tbsp. heavy cream
A pinch of salt
½ cup water
2 tbsps. coconut flour
2 tbsps. flax meal

Directions:
Add the water, salt, coconut flour, and flax meal to a small pot and let it simmer.
Keep whisking until it simmers.
Remove from heat and then add the beaten egg.
Continue whisking until it thickens.
Remove from heat and add the butter, cream, and sweetener.
Garnish with any of your favorite toppings like berries or unsweetened coconut flakes.

Cinnamon Keto Granola

(2 servings total; breakfast)
(Per serving: 183 calories, 16 grams of fat, 8 grams of fiber, 11.8 grams of carbs, 5.9 grams of protein)

Ingredients:
1 oz. mixed nuts like walnuts, almonds, pecans
2 tbsps. flaxseed meal
2 tbsps. coconut flakes, unsweetened
½ tbsp. chia seeds
½ tsp. ground cinnamon
1 tbsp. Stevia® sugar substitute

Directions:
Preheat your oven to 350°F.
Combine all the ingredients in a big bowl.
Spread out the mixture on a parchment-lined baking sheet.
Bake for 20–22 minutes.
Let it cool, and the granola will harden.

Keto Blueberry Pancakes

(1 serving; breakfast)
(463 calories, 15 grams of protein, 42 grams of fat, 8 grams of carbs, 12 grams of fiber)

Ingredients:
3 eggs
¼ cup fresh blueberries
A pinch salt
2 oz. cream cheese
1 tbsp. melted butter
1/3 cup almond flour
1/3 cup oats
1 tsp. baking powder
¼ lemon zest

Directions:
In a bowl, whisk together cream cheese, eggs, and melted butter.
Mix the rest of the ingredients except your blueberries.
Then add the egg mixture to the dry ingredients.
Combine until you get a smooth batter.
You can pour half the batter into a skillet to make a pancake, top with blueberries, and flip to cook the other side.
Use the other half for another.

Raspberry Avocado Smoothie

(1 serving; breakfast)
(208 calories, 20 grams of fat, 13 grams of carbs, 2.7 grams of protein)

Ingredients:
½ avocado, pitted, peeled, and diced
½ cup water
1 tbsp. lemon juice
¼ cup frozen organic raspberries
1–2 tbsp. Stevia® sugar
Directions:
Add all the ingredients to a blender and blend until smooth.

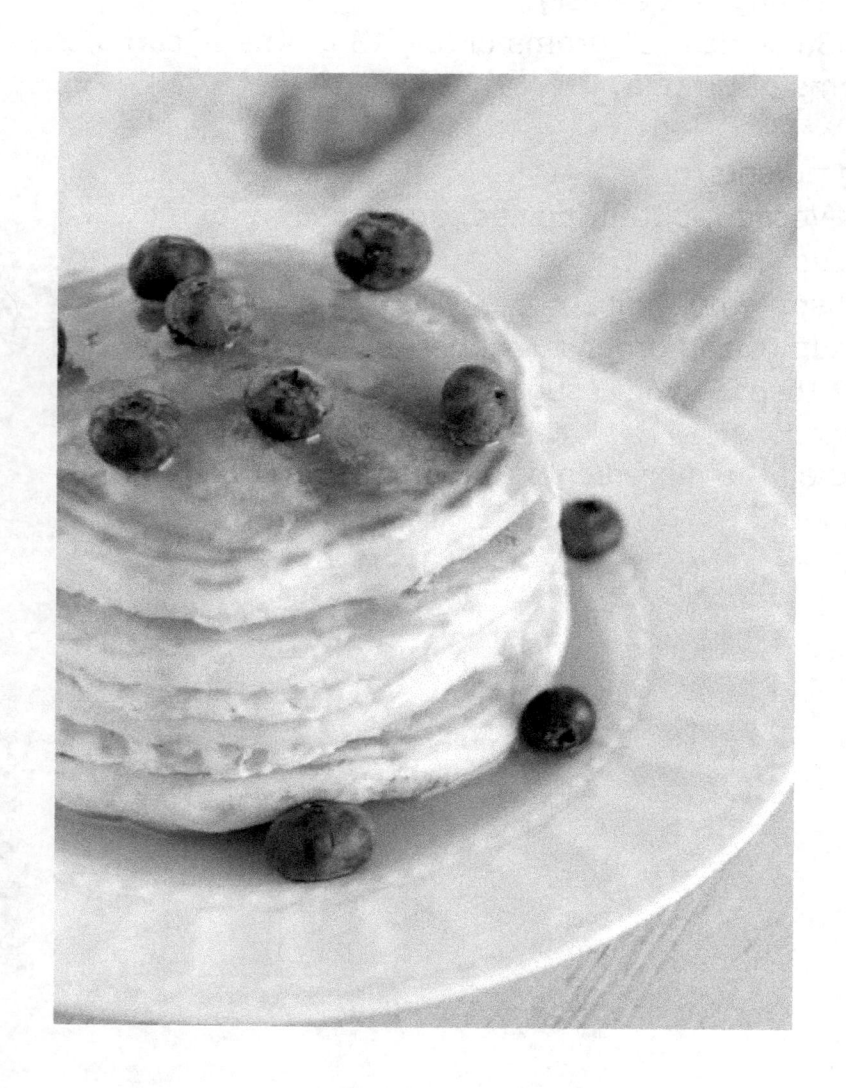

Lunch

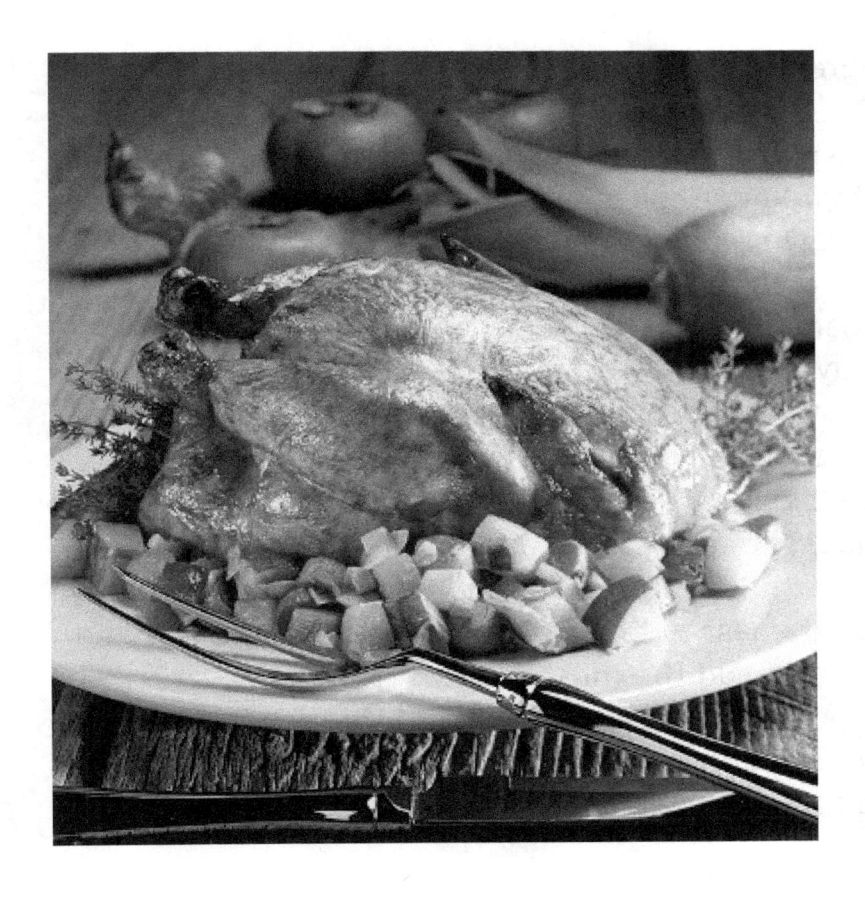

Zucchini and Avocado Noodles

(1 serving; lunch)
(389 calories, 18 grams of carbs, 10 grams of fiber, 5 grams of protein)

Ingredients:
10–15 basil leaves
½ tsp. salt
1 tsp. lemon juice
3 brown mushrooms, sliced
1 ½ tbsp. olive oil
1 garlic clove
½ avocado—pitted and peeled
1 serving zucchini noodles

Directions:
In a blender, add together the avocado, basil, lemon juice, salt, and garlic, and 1 tablespoon olive oil.
Pulse until everything is well-combined and creamy.
Add the last ½ tablespoons of olive oil into a frying pan and add the mushrooms.
Cook until tender and then add the zucchini noodles and cook until they become warm.
Add the avocado sauce and mix together.

BLT Lettuce Wraps

(1 serving; lunch)
(373 calories, 10.6 grams of carbs, 3.4 grams of fiber, 8.9 grams of protein)

Ingredients:
2 lettuce leaves
½ avocado, pitted, peeled, and sliced
1 tbsp. mayo
2 slices bacon
¼ tomato, sliced
1 tsp. olive oil
Directions:
In a saucepan on medium heat, add the olive oil and fry the bacon until it's crispy.
Spoon out some mayo on each lettuce leaf and add the bacon, tomato, and avocado slices.

Rosemary Chicken w/ Broccoli

(1 serving; lunch)
(472 calories, 33 grams of fat, 7 grams of carbs, 34 grams of protein, 2.8 grams of fiber)

Ingredients:
1 boneless chicken breast
1 tbsp. olive oil
2 tbsps. water
½ tsp. rosemary
¼ broccoli head
Salt and pepper to taste

Directions:
Cut the chicken into bite-size pieces.
Season with salt and pepper. Season the broccoli into small florets and season that if you prefer it that way.
In a skillet on medium heat, add the olive oil and cook the chicken with the rosemary. Cook for 3–5 minutes until it turns golden brown and is no longer raw.
Add the broccoli and cook for another few minutes until it's tender.
Add the water and cover the pan so everything can cook together.

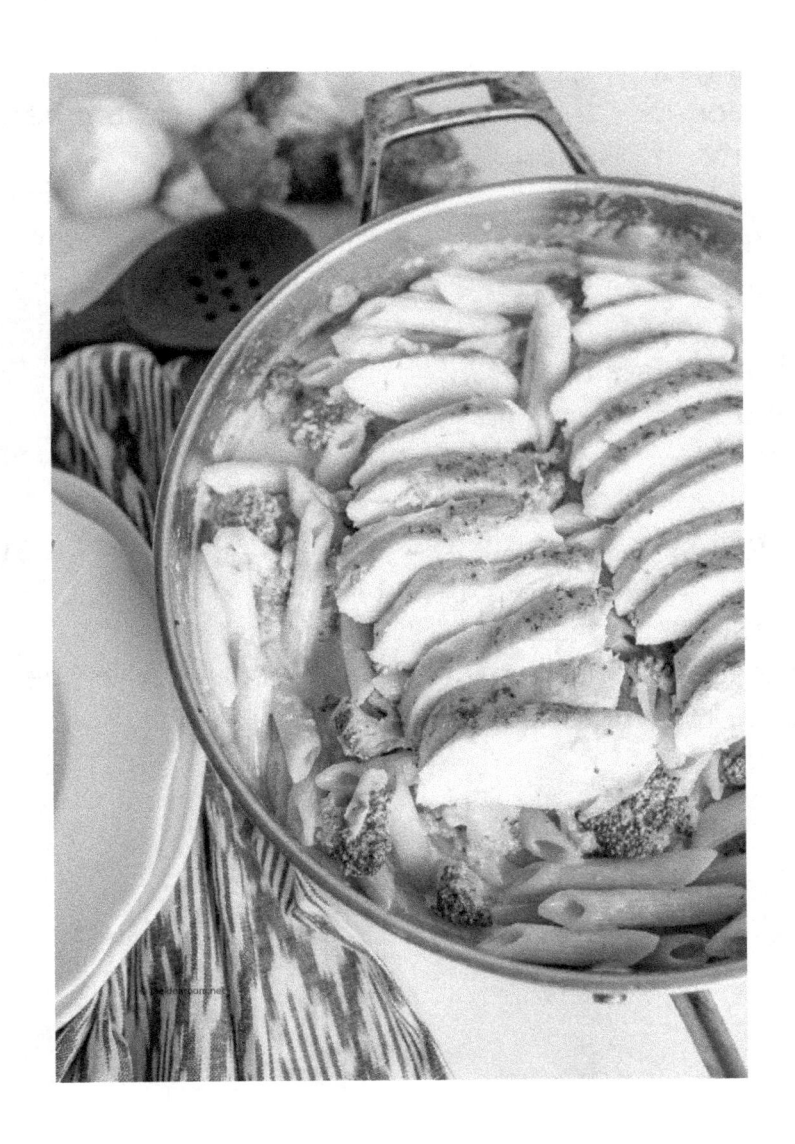

Caesar Salad

(1 serving; lunch)
(210 calories, 7.9 grams of carbs, 2.6 grams of fiber, 8.9 grams of protein)

Ingredients:
4 lettuce leaves
1 tbsp. Caesar dressing
6–8 broccoli stems
½ tomato
1 egg
Directions:
First, boil your egg until it is hard-boiled, however you prefer it. Peel then slice it and keep it aside.
Then boil the broccoli until it is tender.
Tear the lettuce leaves into a bowl and mix with the broccoli, tomato, and egg.
Add the dressing.

Turkey Chili

(2 servings total; lunch)
(1 serving: 390 calories, 27 grams of protein, 31 grams of fat, 8 grams of carbohydrates)

Ingredients:
1 tsp. salt, thyme, black pepper, red chili powder, and garlic powder
1 cup diced onion
3 tbsps. coconut oil
2 cups coconut milk
1-pound organic ground turkey
2-3 garlic cloves, minced

Directions:
In a large pot, heat your coconut oil.
Add the garlic when the oil is hot.
When the garlic becomes fragrant, add your onion and turkey and the spices and stir until well-combined.
Stir until the turkey is golden brown.
Add the coconut milk and bring to a boil. Keep stirring to avoid burning.
Reduce the heat for 10–15 minutes, then remove from heat.

Deli Meat Plate

(2 servings total; lunch)
(1 serving: 22 calories, 40 grams of protein, 59 grams of fat, 3 grams of fiber, 11 grams of carbs, 8 grams of net carbs)

Ingredients:
Salt and pepper to taste
¼ cup olive oil
2 tomatoes, sliced
2 garlic cloves, minced
10 green or black olives
7 oz. prosciutto, sliced
7 oz. mozzarella cheese

Directions:
In a plate, lay out your cheese, prosciutto, olives, and tomatoes.
Sprinkle with salt, pepper, minced garlic, and olive oil.

Kale Beef and Veggie Wrap

(1 serving; lunch)
(731 calories, 60 grams of fat, 17 grams of fat, 30 grams of protein)

Ingredients:
2 large kale leaves
½ avocado, pitted, peeled, and sliced
½ tomato, sliced
100 grams ground beef
1 tbsp. olive oil
½ tsp. salt, pepper, and chili powder

Directions:
Trim the stem of the kale leaf so you can fold the leaf as if it's the bread of a sandwich.
Slice your avocado and tomato.
Season the ground beef with salt, pepper, and chili powder.
In a saucepan on medium heat, add the olive oil, then fry the ground beef until cooked through.
Divide the ground beef into each kale leaf and add the vegetable toppings.
Carefully wrap the kale leaf around the meat and veggies and use an aluminum foil to hold it tight.

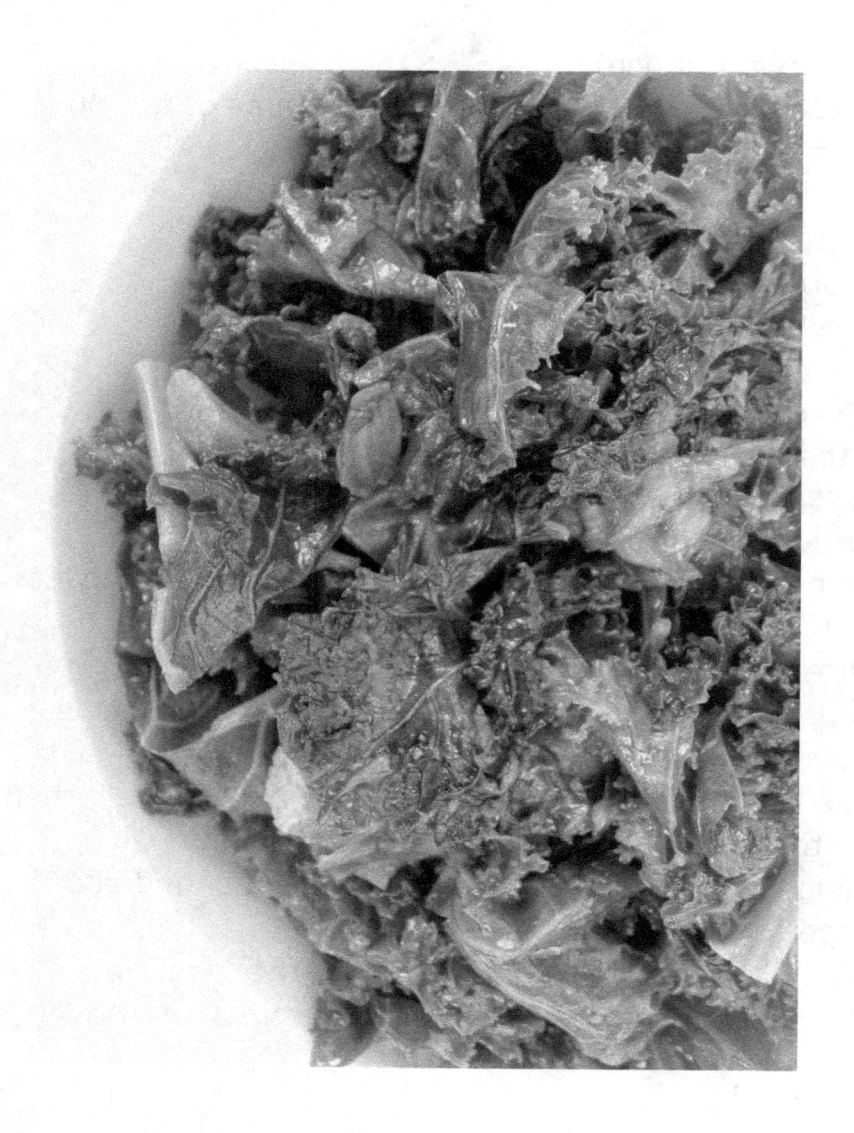

Keto Crescent Hot Dogs

(8 hot dogs; lunch)
(Per serving: 349 calories, 29 grams of fat, 8 grams of carbs, 18 grams of protein)

Ingredients:
8 large hot dogs
1 egg
¾ cup almond flour
1-ounce cream cheese
1.75 grated mozzarella cheese
Directions:
Preheat your oven to 400°F.
In a large mixing bowl, add the almond flour, cheese, and cream cheese.
Microwave for 30 seconds until the cheese becomes soft.
Add the egg and mix everything together until it forms a dough-like mixture.
Divide the dough into 8 portions.
On wax paper or parchment paper, roll out the dough into a rectangle.
Carefully wrap the dough around the hot dog like a spiral formation.
Bake for 20–30 minutes until the dough becomes golden brown.

Keto Friendly Pizza Rolls

(3 servings total; lunch)
(1 serving: 127 calories, 3 grams of carbs, 8 grams of fat, 11 grams of protein, 1 gram of fiber)

Ingredients:
½ tsp. pizza seasoning
¼ cup meat topping of your choice like crumbled sausage or pepperoni slices
1 cup mozzarella cheese
½ cup low-carb pizza sauce
¼ cup tomatoes, sliced
2 tbsps. White onion, diced
¼ cup bell peppers, chopped

Directions:
First, preheat your oven to 400°F and line a baking sheet with parchment paper.
Sprinkle out the cheese all over the pan in a single layer and make sure there aren't any holes or gaps in the layer.
Sprinkle the pizza seasoning.
Bake for 15 minutes or until the cheese turns golden brown.
Remove from the oven and add your topping of meat, bell pepper, onions, and tomato slices.
Drizzle the pizza sauce all over.
Bake in the oven again for another 15 minutes or until the top is golden brown.

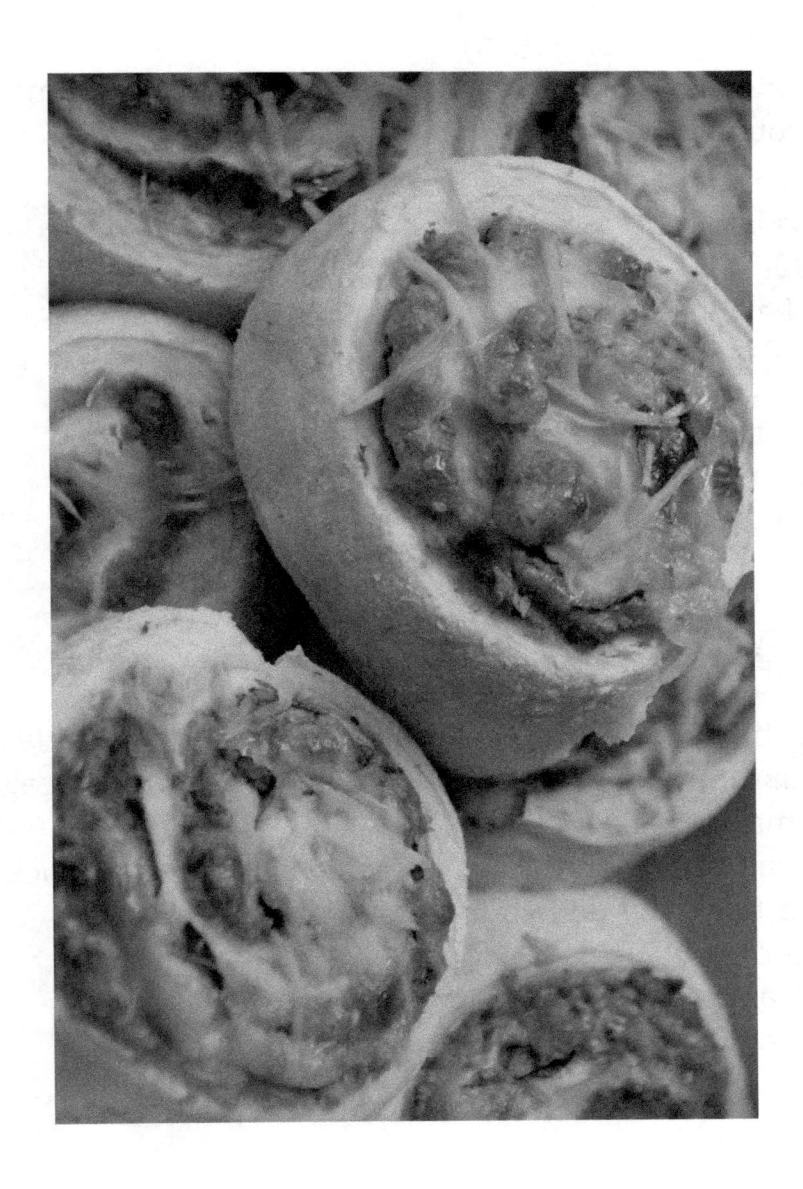

Tuna Salad and Boiled Eggs

(2 servings total; lunch)
(1 serving: 405 calories, 6 grams of carbs, 21 grams of protein, 2 grams of fiber)

Ingredients:
4 eggs
2 cups shredded lettuce
2 tbsps. onion, diced
1 tbsp. sour cream
1 can tuna
Salt and pepper to taste
1 tbsp. mayonnaise
½ tomato, sliced
1 tsp. lemon juice
1 tsp. olive oil
Directions:
First, boil your eggs, peel, halve them, and set aside.
In a large bowl, mix together your tuna, lemon juice, and mayonnaise.
Add salt and pepper to your taste. Shred your lettuce into a bowl and add your onions, sour cream, and tomato slices.
Then add the tuna mixture.
Drizzle with olive oil as a dressing.

20 Minute Meatballs

(8 servings total; lunch)
(1 serving: 63 calories, 10 grams of fat, 1 gram of carbs, 12 grams of protein)

Ingredients:
1-pound ground beef
1 tsp. salt
1 tsp. black pepper
1 tbsp. minced garlic
1 large egg
½ cup grated parmesan
½ cup shredded mozzarella

Directions:
Preheat your oven to 400°F.
In a large bowl, mix together all the ingredients until well-combined.
Form about 16 evenly-sized meatballs and place them on a parchment-lined baking sheet.
Bake for 18–20 minutes or until golden brown.

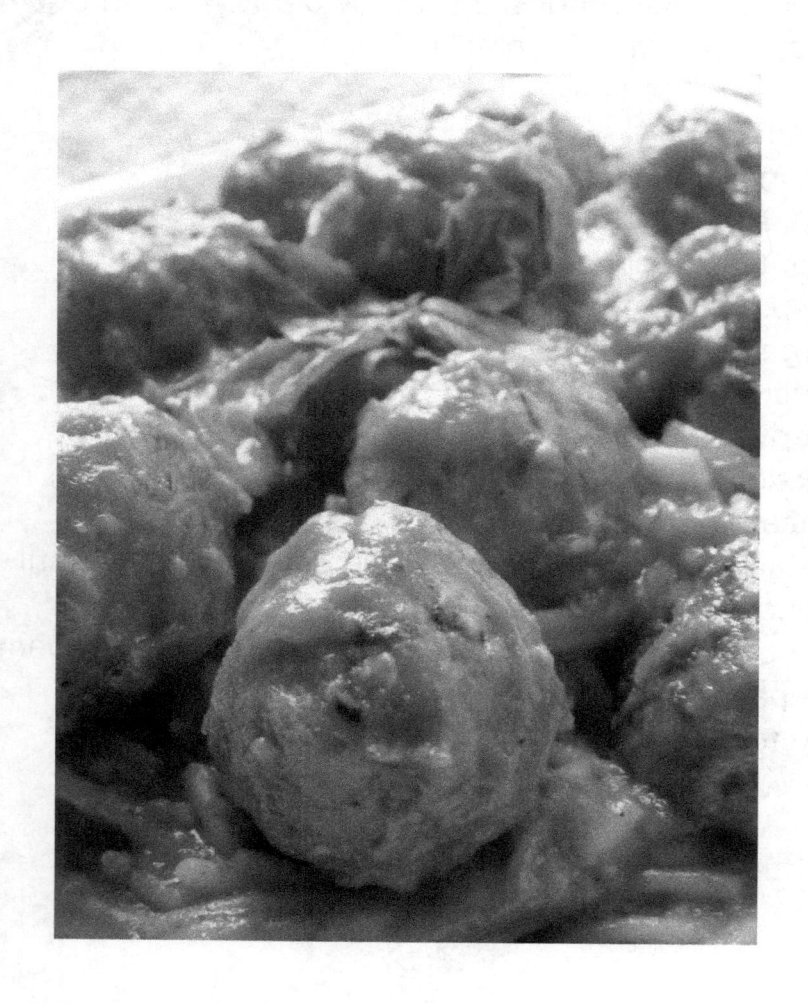

Avocado Egg Salad

(6 servings total; lunch)
(Per serving: 159 calories, 12 grams of fat, 8 grams of protein, 4 grams of fiber, 8 grams of carbs)

Ingredients:
1 tsp. dried herbs
½ tsp. salt
½ tsp. black pepper
¼ cup onion, minced
2 tbsps. lemon juice
2 avocados, pitted, peeled, and diced
6 hard-boiled eggs

Directions:
Peel your hard-boiled eggs and place them in a large mixing bowl.
Add your avocado and mash and combine the two ingredients, so the avocado coats the eggs.
Add the lemon juice, onion, herbs, and salt and pepper.
Stir well.

Chicken Cucumber Avocado Salad

(3 servings total; lunch)
(Per serving: 272 calories, 19 grams of fat, 5 grams of carbs, 2.5 grams of fiber, 20 grams of protein)

Ingredients:
1 ½ cup shredded chicken
2 tomatoes, chopped
3 tbsps. lemon juice
Salt and pepper to taste
3 tbsps. olive oil
¼ fresh parsley, chopped
1 avocado, pitted, peeled, diced
¼ cup onion, sliced
1 large cucumber, diced
Directions:
In a large bowl, mix the chicken, cucumber, tomatoes, avocado, onion, and parsley.
Drizzle with lemon juice and olive oil.
Season with salt and pepper.
Mix to combine everything.

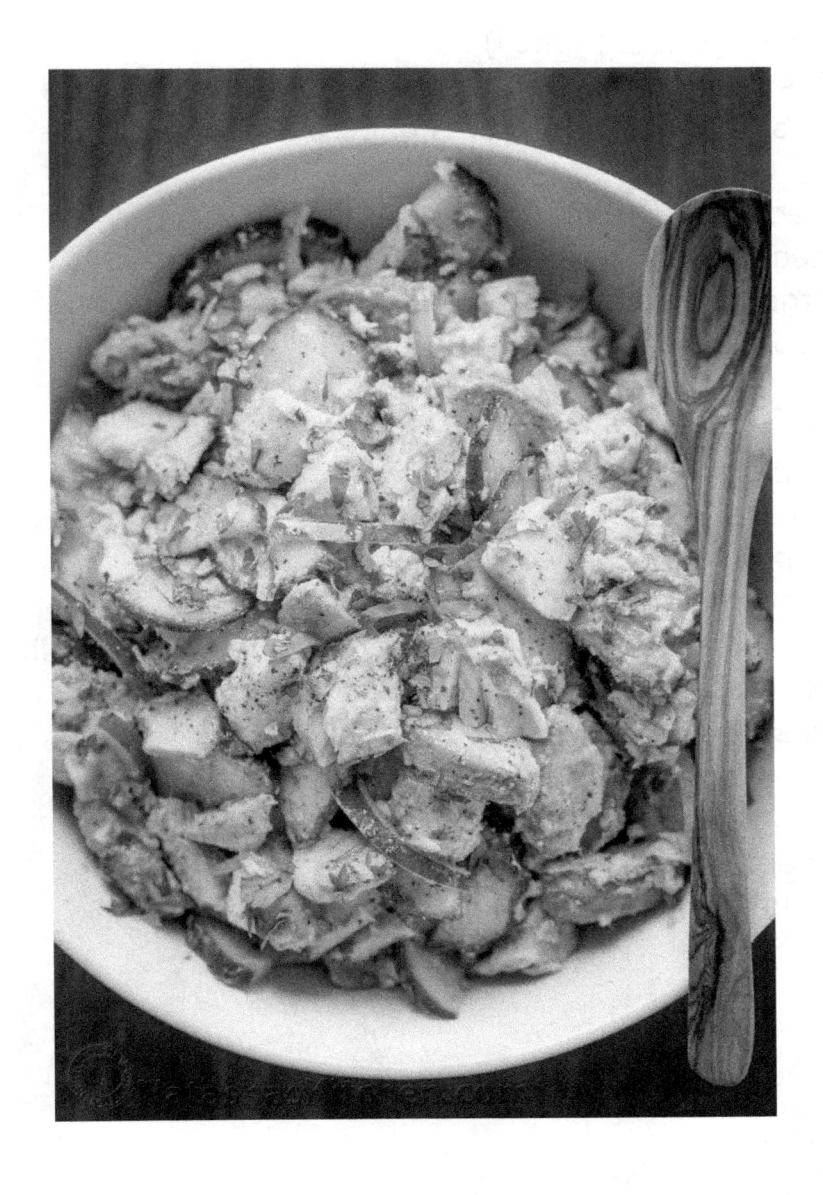

Sesame Salad

(6 servings total; lunch)
(Per serving total: 375 calories, 26 grams of fat, 24 grams of protein, 16 grams of carbs)

Ingredients:
1 medium lettuce head, chopped
2 large salmon filets (~12 ounces each)
4 tbsps. olive oil
1 tsp. sesame oil
¼ cup green onions, chopped
1 medium bell pepper, chopped
1 tomato, chopped
¼ cup onion, chopped
Directions:
In a saucepan on medium heat, heat up the olive oil. If you want, you can cut your salmon into smaller pieces. Then, let it cook.
Flip it over and cook the other side. When done cooking, place in a bowl with your chopped lettuce, peppers, tomato, and onion.
Add the sesame oil as a salad dressing.

Keto Tuna Salad

(1 serving; lunch)
(285 calories, 24 grams of fat, 2 grams of fiber, 20 grams of protein, 3 grams of carbs)

Ingredients:
3 slices bacon
1 hard-boiled egg
1 tbsp. olive oil
1 can tuna (~14 ounces)
2 tbsps. onion, chopped
1 tbsp. sour cream
2 tsp. Dijon mustard
½ tsp. dried herbs
1 tbsp. mayonnaise
Directions:
In a saucepan on medium heat, add the olive oil and cook the bacon.
Drain the tuna and add to a large bowl along with the chopped onion and hard-boiled egg.
Add the other ingredients and the herbs and top with the crumbled bacon.

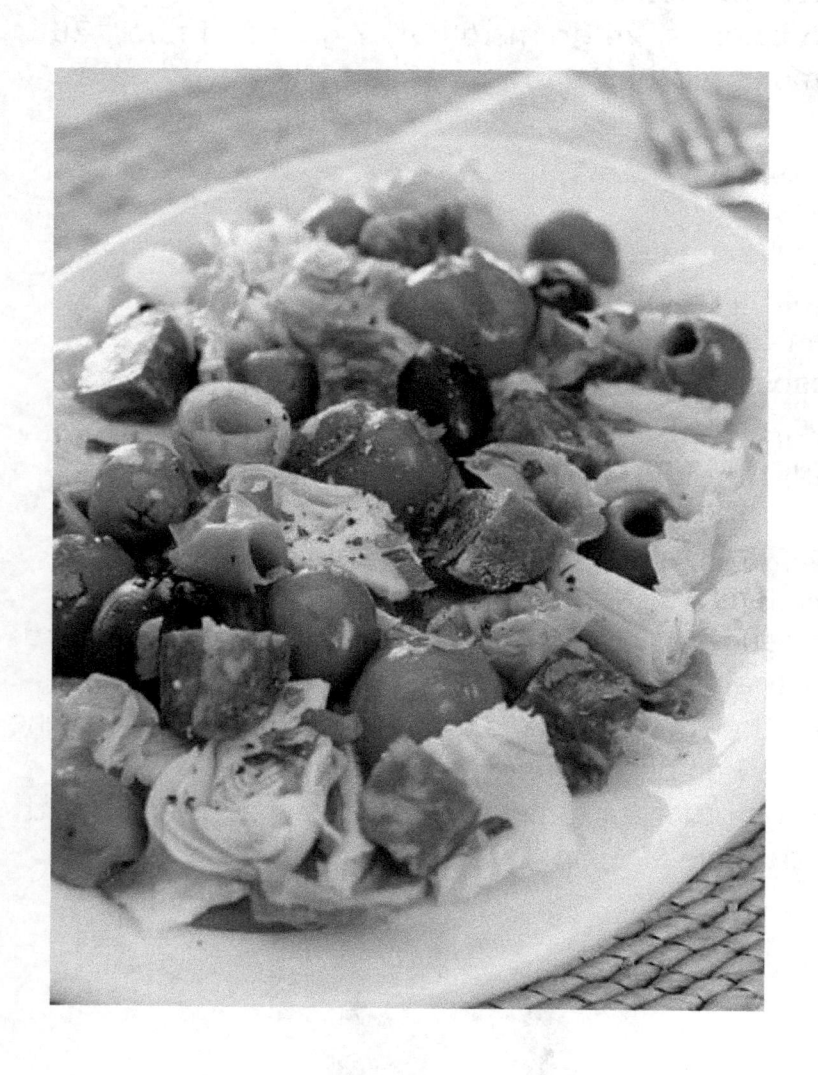

Pesto Chicken Salad

(4 servings total; lunch)
(Per serving: 383 calories, 29 grams of fat, 25 grams of protein, 18 grams of carbs)

Ingredients:
1-pound chicken, cooked and shredded
¼ cup tomato, diced
2 tbsps. green pesto
1 avocado, pitted, peeled, sliced
8–10 slices bacon, cooked and crumbled
1 tsp. olive oil
Salt and pepper to taste
Directions:
In a large mixing bowl, combine all your ingredients. Season with salt and pepper and add olive oil as a dressing.

Low-Carb Chicken Nuggets

(3 servings total; lunch)
(Per serving: 223 calories, 16.4 grams of fat, 2 grams of carbs, 17.2 grams of protein)

Ingredients:
1 cup cooked chicken
1 egg
2 garlic cloves, minced
¼ cup almond flour
4 oz. grass-fed cream cheese
Directions:
Preheat your oven to 350°F.
Then, shred the chicken. This recipe works best if it's warm so that you can microwave it for a minute.
Once shredded, combined with the other ingredients. Make about 10 evenly sized balls and place them on a parchment-lined baking sheet.
Bake for 12–15 minutes until golden brown.

Taco Casserole

(3 servings total; lunch)
(Per serving: 354 calories, 6 grams of carbs, 43 grams of protein, 18 grams of fat)

Ingredients:
½ cup salsa
8 oz. cottage cheese
4 oz. shredded cheddar cheese
Salt and pepper to taste
1 tbsp. taco seasoning
¾ cup ground beef

Directions:
Preheat your oven to 400°F.
In a large casserole dish, mix the ground beef with the taco seasoning.
Bake for 15 minutes.
In another bowl, mix the salsa, 1 cup of cheddar, and cottage cheese.
Spread the cottage cheese mixture on top of the meat and sprinkle with the remaining cheese.
Bake for another 15–20 minutes until cooked thoroughly.

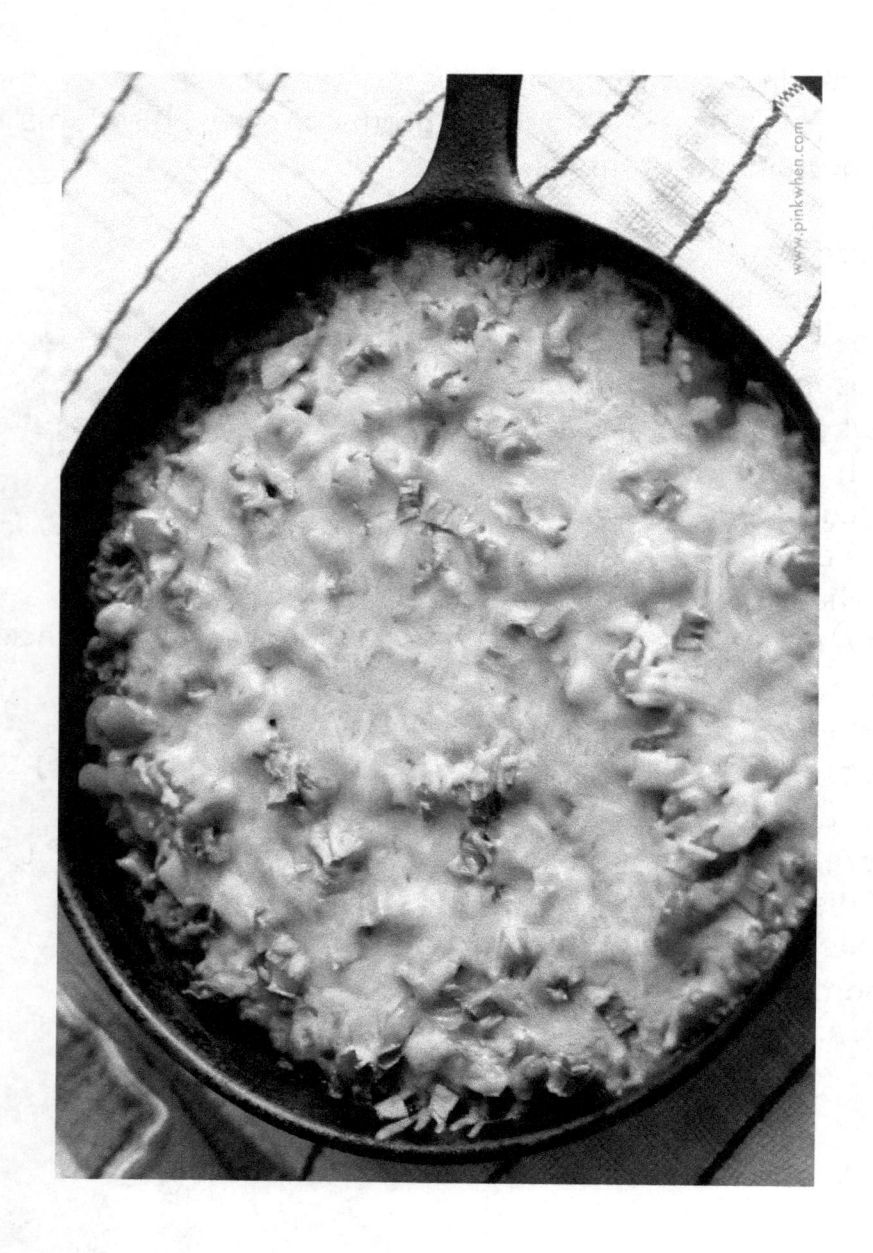

Tomato Basil Soup

(3 servings total; lunch)
(Per serving: 284 calories, 29 grams of fat, 6.3 grams of carbs, 1 gram of fiber, 3 grams of fiber)

Ingredients:
2 ½ cups fresh tomato puree (you can use a blender to blend your tomatoes)
4 oz. cream cheese
A handful basil leaves
4 tbsps. butter
1 tbsp. Stevia® sugar sweetener
Salt and pepper to taste
Directions:
Once you have your tomatoes pureed, add to a large saucepan with the butter and cream.
Heat to a simmer and cook until thick. Turn off the heat and once cool, add to your blender with your basil leaves and sweetener and blend until smooth—season with salt and pepper.

Chocolate Coconut Keto Smoothie

(1 serving; lunch)
(500 calories, 29 grams of protein, 3 grams of fiber, 12 grams of carbs)

Ingredients:
¾ cup full-fat coconut milk
A handful ice
2 scoops protein powder
15–20 drops liquid coconut Stevia® (or plain Stevia®)
2 tbsps. cacao powder, unsweetened
Directions:
Add all the ingredients except the protein powder into a blender and blend well.
Add the protein powder and blend gently.
Enjoy immediately or chill for a half-hour if you enjoy a cold treat with a thicker consistency.

Cheesy Bacon Chicken

(3 servings total; lunch)
(Per serving: 321 calories, 21 grams of fat, 29.1 grams of protein, 1 gram carbs)

Ingredients:
3 chicken breasts
½ cup shredded cheddar cheese
8–10 bacon strips
1 tsp. barbeque seasoning
Salt and pepper to taste
Directions:
Preheat your oven to 400°F.
Rub both sides of the chicken breasts with the seasoning and salt and pepper.
Top each piece with a few pieces of bacon.
Bake for 30 minutes until the bacon is crispy and the chicken is almost cooked through.
Remove the tray and sprinkle with the cheese.
Bake for another 10–15 minutes until the cheese is bubbly.
Serve with low-carb barbecue sauce.

Dinner

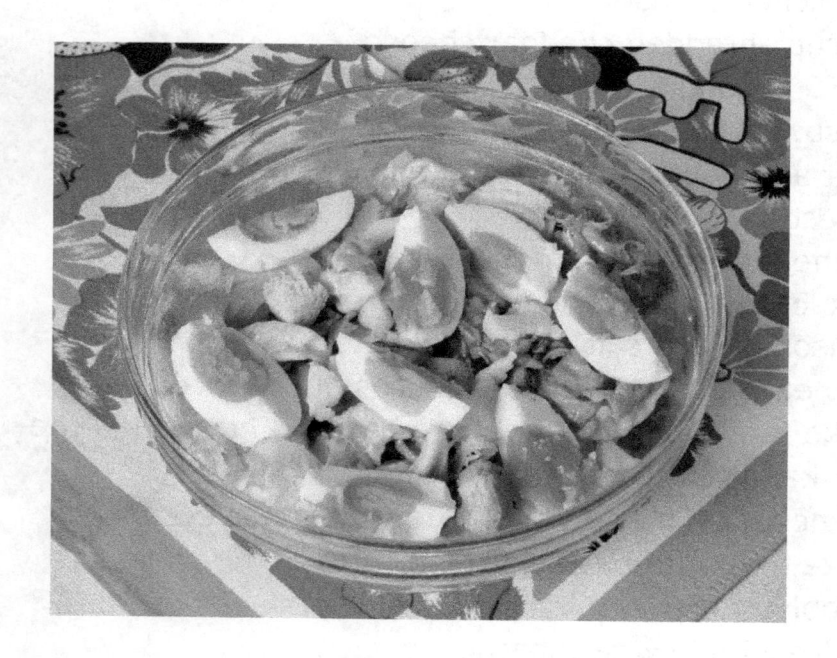

Steak Stir Fry

(4 servings total; dinner)
(290 calories per serving, 14 grams of fat, 38.2 grams of protein, 13 grams of carbs)

Ingredients:
1 small bell pepper, sliced
1 small onion, sliced
¼ cup mushrooms, sliced
1 cup beef broth
1 tsp. ginger, minced
2 garlic cloves, minced
1 tbsp. olive oil
1-pound beef sirloin
2 tbsps. low-carb soy sauce
Salt and pepper to taste
Directions:
Add the olive oil to a large skillet over medium heat. Once hot, add the beef and crumble it in the pan.
Add ginger and garlic to let it season. Let it brown for about 5 minutes on each side until fragrant—season with salt and pepper. Remove from heat.
Add the peppers, onions, and mushroom. Stir the vegetables until soft for about 3–5 minutes.
Add the soy sauce and beef broth, then return the beef to the pan to cook.
Let simmer for a few minutes until some of the liquid evaporates, then remove from heat.

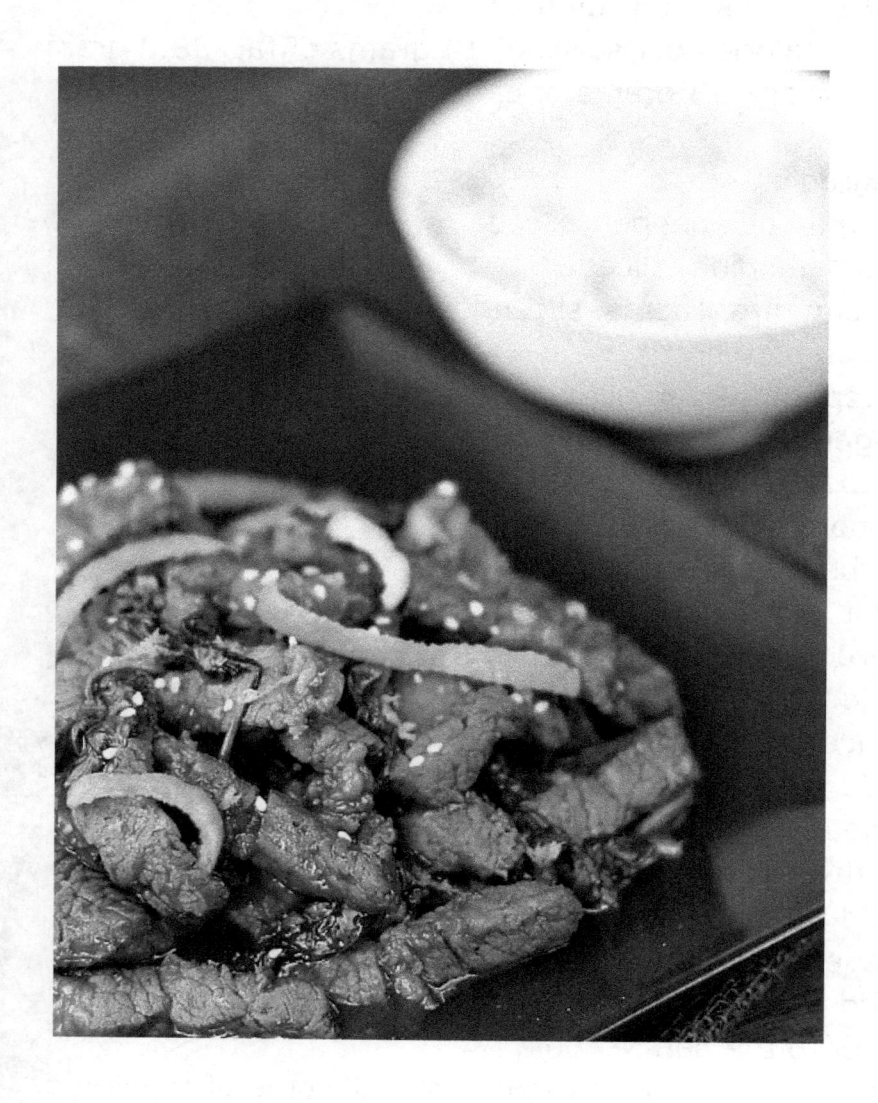

Grilled Shrimp & Cod Fillet

(2 servings total; dinner)
(348 calories, 5.5 grams of carbs, 1 gram of fiber, 55.9 grams of protein)

Ingredients:
2 cod fillets
8-10 cherry tomatoes
3 garlic cloves, minced
1 tbsp. lemon juice
200 grams shrimp
1 tbsp. fresh parsley, finely chopped
1 tbsp. butter
Salt and pepper to taste
Directions:
In a saucepan on medium heat, melt the butter.
Add the minced garlic, and once fragrant, add the fish and shrimp to the pan.
For the codfish, cook for 2-3 minutes on each side—season with salt and pepper to your taste. Be gentle when flipping, so it doesn't break apart.
Add the tomatoes and cook until soft.
Add the lemon juice and fresh parsley on top as a garnish.

Arugula Caesar Salad

(1 serving; dinner)
(273 calories, 19 grams of carbs, 9 grams of fiber, 7 grams of protein)

Ingredients:
1 stalk of arugula (~40 grams)
3 leaves iceberg lettuce
6–7 slices cucumber
½ avocado, pitted, peeled, and sliced
½ tomato, sliced
4–5 broccoli florets
2 asparagus
Directions:
First, boil the asparagus and broccoli until they are tender.
Shred the lettuce and arugula and put them into the bowl.
Add the avocado, tomato, and cucumber slices.
Toss together and season with Caesar dressing.

Rosemary Pork Roast

(3 servings total; dinner)
(1 serving: 367 calories, 0.12 grams of carbs, 0.3 grams of fiber, 33.8 grams of protein)

Ingredients:
500 grams boneless pork roast
1 tsp. black pepper
1 tsp. salt
1 tbsp. olive oil
1 tsp. red chili powder
1 tbsp. rosemary, finely chopped
Directions:
Preheat your oven to 400°F.
Season your pork roast with olive oil, salt, pepper, and rosemary.
Massage it in well and let marinate for 20–30 minutes.
Place on a baking sheet lined with parchment paper—
Bake for 1 hour. You can pan-fry on the stove if you want extra char.

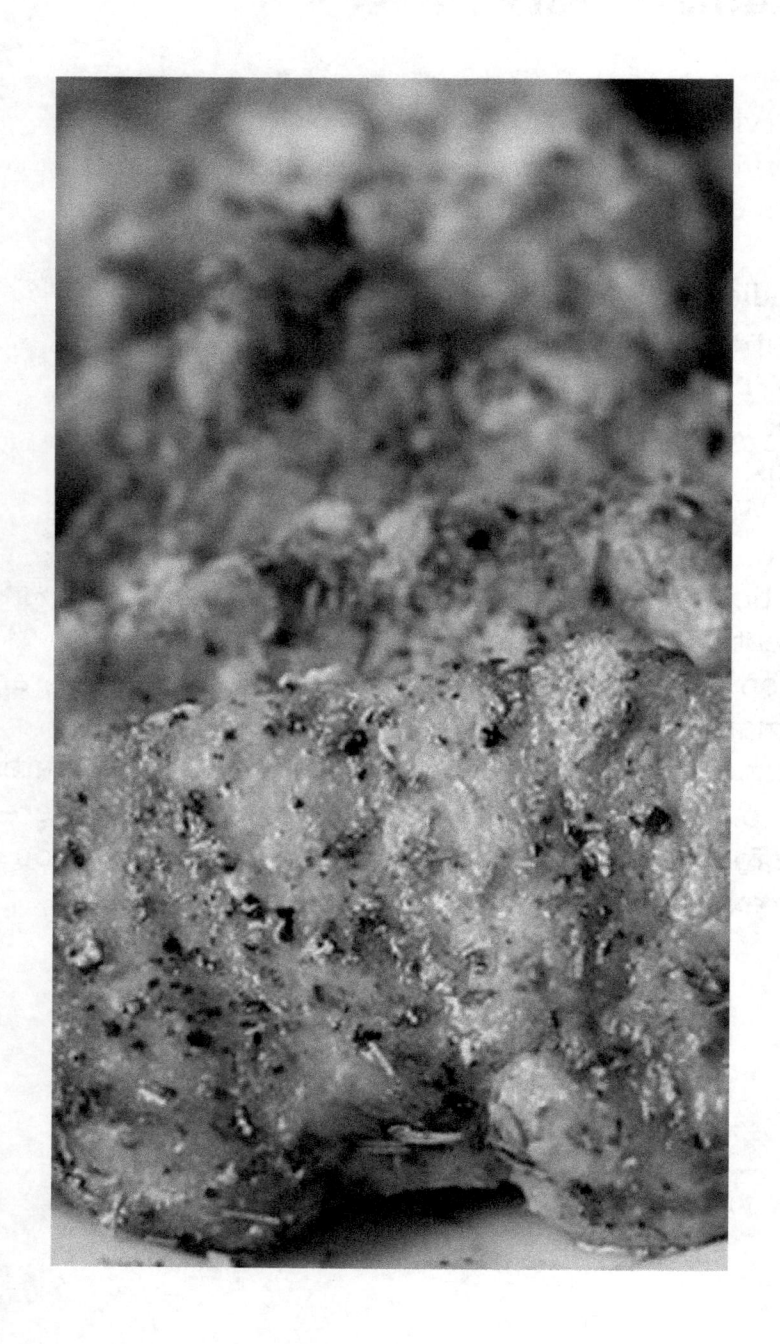

Broccoli and Bacon with Mushrooms

(1 serving; dinner)
(382 calories, 4 grams of carbs, 1.8 grams of fiber, 32 grams of protein)

Ingredients:
¼ broccoli stalk
4 brown mushrooms
8–10 slices bacon
1 tbsp. olive oil
¼ tsp. salt
¼ tsp. pepper
¼ tsp. garlic powder
¼ tsp. rosemary
Water
Directions:
Put water to boil and cook the broccoli until it's tender.
In a saucepan on medium heat, add the olive oil and fry the bacon until golden brown.
Slice the mushrooms and season with salt and pepper, and add to the pan.
Add the rosemary and garlic powder and fry with the bacon and mushrooms. Mix everything together.

Lettuce Burger

(1 serving; dinner)
(378 calories, 2.9 grams of carbs, 1.3 grams of fiber, 16 grams of protein)

Ingredients:
40 grams ground beef (about enough for 1 hamburger patty)
1 large lettuce leaf
1 cup baby spinach
2 slices bacon
2-3 slices tomato
1 tbsp. mayo
Salt and pepper to taste
Directions:
In a saucepan, fry the bacon first until it is golden brown.
Mix salt and pepper to the ground beef and form a hamburger patty shape and fry in the leftover bacon grease. Cook both sides until golden brown, then remove from heat.
Add the spinach to the pan and cook until wilted. Season with salt and pepper as necessary.
Add the mayo, tomato, patty, bacon, and spinach to the large lettuce leaf. Fold and eat like a burger.

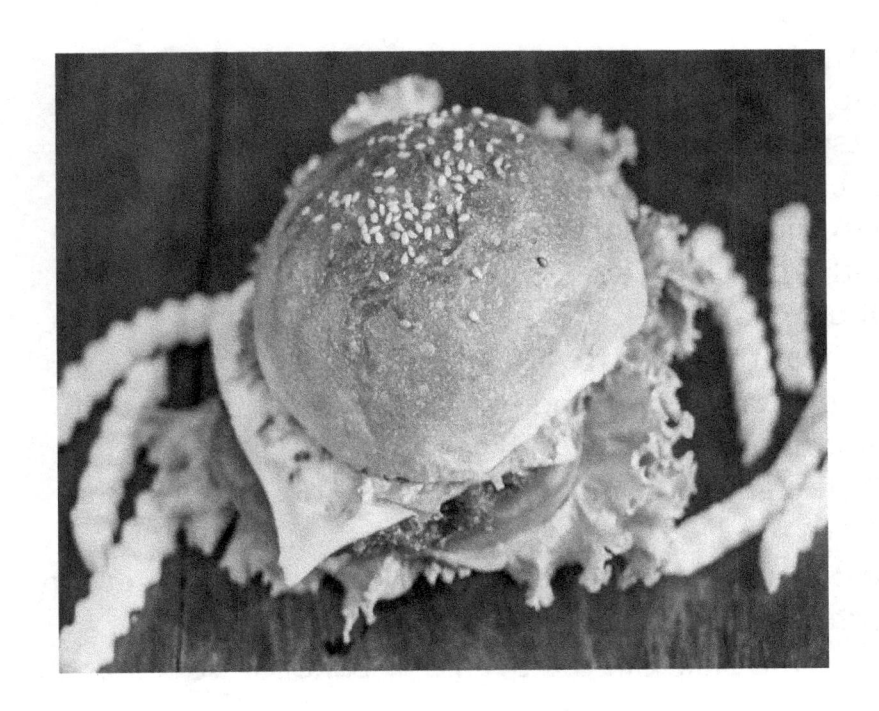

Roasted Chicken Leg with Veggies

(2 servings total; dinner)
(Per serving: 635 calories, 38 grams of fat, 9 grams of carbs, 3 grams of fiber, 64 grams of protein)

Ingredients:
8–10 baby carrots
2 chicken legs
6–8 cherry tomatoes
1 tsp. salt, pepper, cumin powder, red chili powder
1 tbsp. olive oil
6–8 slices zucchini
6–8 broccoli florets
Directions:
Preheat the oven to 400°F.
Slice your veggies and fry in a saucepan on medium heat until soft.
Then place on a lined baking sheet or in a cast-iron skillet.
Add the chicken legs to the tray or skillet and season with the spices, and massage in the olive oil.
Place the skillet in the oven and bake for 50 minutes.

Grilled Chicken with Guacamole

(1 serving; dinner)
(632 calories, 15 grams of carbs, 8.9 grams of fiber, 41.8 grams of protein)

Ingredients:
2 tbsps. olive oil
½ tsp. salt, pepper, chili powder
1 chicken thigh with skin
½ avocado—pitted and peeled
¼ tomato
1 slice red onion

Directions:
Marinate the chicken with salt, pepper, and half the olive oil.
Heat the rest of the olive oil in a cast-iron skillet and place the chicken with the skin side down.
Grill both sides until cooked, about 4–6 minutes each side. Dice the tomato and red onion.
Mash the avocado and mix with the tomato and red onion, and season with salt and pepper.
Top over the chicken.

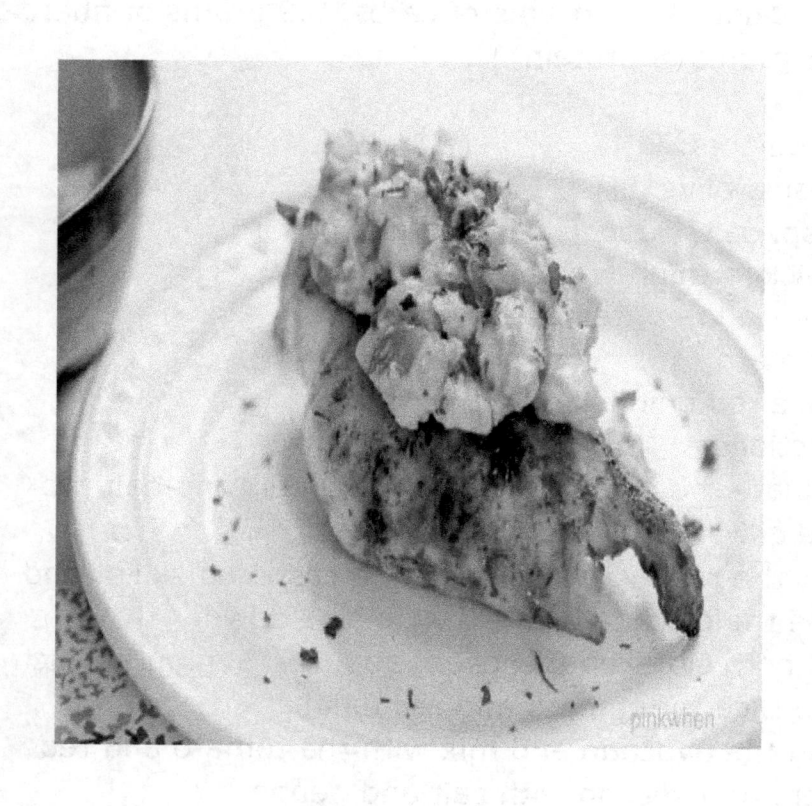

Grilled Salmon and Green Beans

(1 serving; dinner)
(389 calories, 9.02 grams of carbs, 2.7 grams of fiber, 32.08 grams of protein)

Ingredients:
1 salmon fillet (~150 grams)
3 tbsps. olive oil in 3 portions
1 tsp. salt, pepper, and dill
1 tsp. lemon juice
1 tbsp. rosemary
5–6 small radishes
1 cup green beans
2 garlic cloves, minced

Directions:
Marinate the salad with the oil, salt, and pepper.
Add a tablespoon of olive oil to a frying pan and cook the fish on both sides for 3–4 minutes until cooked through.
Add the lemon juice over the salmon once you remove it from the heat.
Boil the green beans until they are soft.
Then add to the frying pan along with the garlic and sprinkle with salt and pepper until cooked.
Add the radishes and rosemary to the pan and fry until crispy.
Sprinkle with salt and pepper.

Serve everything together on a plate.

Mexican Cauliflower Rice

(3 servings total; dinner)
(1 serving: 103 calories, 5.8 grams of fat, 12 grams of carbs, 3 grams of protein)

Ingredients:
3 cup cauliflower rice
1 small onion, finely chopped
1 jalapeño, finely chopped
1 tomato, finely chopped
2–3 garlic cloves, minced
2 tbsps. olive oil
1 cup bell pepper, diced
1 tsp. paprika powder, salt, cumin powder, and black pepper
1 tsp. lime juice

Directions:
Make your cauliflower, if you have a head of cauliflower, or you can buy it pre-made.
In a large saucepan, add olive oil to the pan.
Add the garlic, tomatoes, onions, and jalapeño pepper.
Add the spices. Stir-fry for a few minutes until the garlic becomes fragrant, and the tomatoes soften.
Add the bell peppers and the cauliflower rice to the pan and fry until it's tender.
Top with lemon juice and remove from heat.

Creamy Mushroom Chicken

(2 servings total; dinner)
(1 serving: 335 calories, 28 grams of fat, 3 grams of carbs, 24 grams of protein)

Ingredients:
1 small onion, sliced
5–6 cremini mushrooms
2 boneless chicken cutlets
1 tsp. Himalayan salt
1 tsp. black pepper
½ tsp. dried thyme
1/3 cup coconut milk, full-fat
3 tbsps. full-fat butter

Directions:
Heat a skillet on medium heat.
Once hot, add two tablespoons of the butter.
When melted, add in the sliced mushrooms and onions and sprinkle with salt for seasoning.
Sauté until golden brown, then remove from heat.
Add the last tablespoon of butter and add the chicken cutlets into the pan.
Sprinkle with salt, pepper, and thyme.
Cook for 4–5 minutes, and then flip the chicken to cook the other side for another 5 minutes.
Add the mushroom and onion mix back to the pan and pour the coconut milk on top. Let it simmer for a few minutes, then remove from heat.

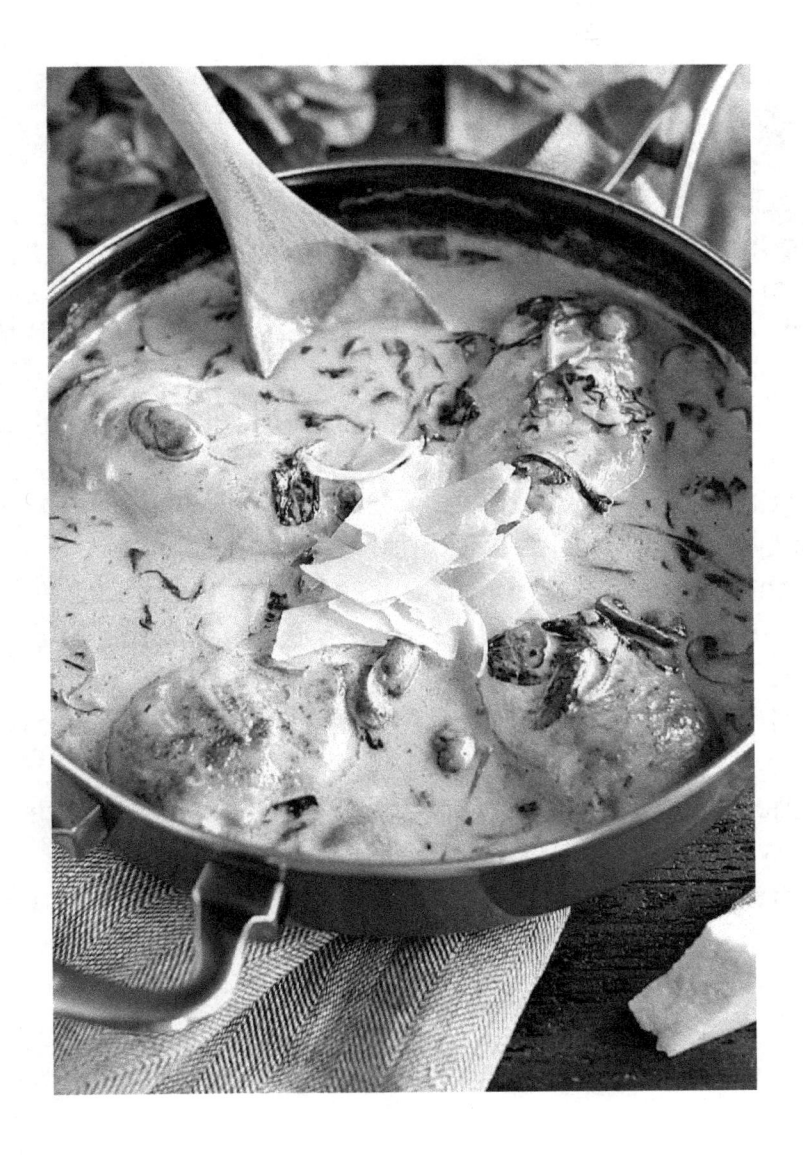

Mushroom Bacon Skillet

(1 serving; dinner)
(233 calories, 8.9 grams of fat, 9.2 grams of carbs, 0.4 grams of fiber, 18 grams of protein)

Ingredients:
6 medium slices bacon
Salt and pepper to taste
1 tsp. garlic powder
1 tsp. olive oil
2 cups mushrooms, halved (either shiitake, cremini, or ali'i all work great)
Directions:
Heat a large skillet on medium heat.
Add the olive oil when hot, and add the bacon slices to the pan. Cook until golden brown, then crumble the pieces and remove from heat.
Add the mushrooms and sauté until golden brown and soft.
Add garlic powder, salt, and pepper to taste and stir until well-combined.
Add the bacon back to the pan and allow it to warm up.
Combine everything together and then remove from heat.

Stuffed Peppers

(6 servings total; dinner)
(Per serving: 169 calories, 5 grams of fat, 27 grams of carbs, 7 grams of protein)

Ingredients:
1 ½ cups marinara sauce
1 pound and 4 oz. ground beef
1 tsp. paprika
1 onion, diced
6 pieces medium to large bell peppers
2 garlic cloves, minced
½ tsp. dried herbs
¼ cup fresh parsley, finely chopped
Salt and pepper to taste
½ cup shredded cheddar cheese
Directions:
Preheat your oven to 375°F.
Add the marinara sauce into a large skillet.
Trim a little of the bottom off each bell pepper, so it sits flat.
Cut off the tops as well and remove the seeds and ribs. In a large bowl, mix the ground beef with the diced onion, paprika, salt and pepper, dried herbs, parsley, and garlic.
Divide the meat mixture into each pepper, filling almost full.
Arrange the peppers in the pan, so they stand in the sauce.
Garnish the peppers with the shredded cheese.

Cook for about 30 minutes until the peppers become soft.
Serve with a scoop of the marinara sauce.
Cauliflower and Bacon Soup (3 servings total; dinner)
(Per serving: 175 calories, 14 grams of fat, 8.5 grams of protein, 19 grams of carbs)

Ingredients:
3 tbsps. olive oil
2-3 tbsps. bacon bits
¾ cup shredded cheddar cheese
½ tsp. xanthan gum (or cornstarch)
¼ cup heavy whipping cream
½ cup water
1 cup chicken broth
½ medium head of cauliflower, chopped
1 tsp. garlic, minced
Directions:
In a large saucepan, heat about 3/4 of the olive oil. Add in the garlic. Once fragrant, add the cauliflower. Pour in the water and chicken broth. Bring to a boil and keep stirring to avoid burning.
Once it's boiling, stir in the heavy cream and reduce the heat.
In a separate bowl, whisk together the rest of the olive oil with the xanthan gum or corn starch to make a thickening paste.
Drop that paste into the soup and stir, so the mixture thickens.
Add in the cheese slowly and stir, so it melts.
Garnish with the bacon.

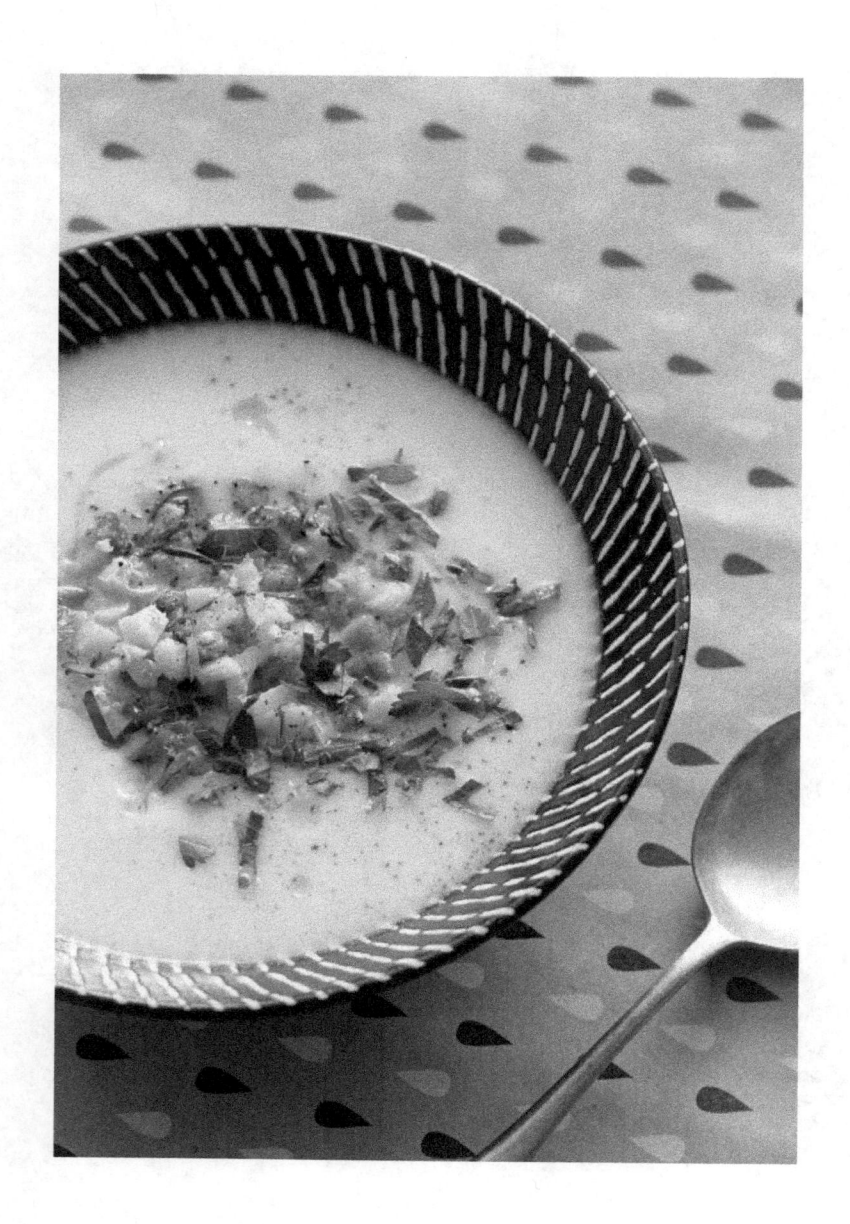

Cabbage Soup

(5 servings total; dinner)
(Per serving: 273 calories, 18 grams of fat, 2 grams of fiber, 6 grams of carbs, 17 grams of protein)
Ingredients:
1-pound ground beef
¼ cup onion, diced
Salt and pepper to taste
1 tsp. cumin powder
½ head cabbage, chopped
2 cups beef broth
1 tbsp. olive oil
2 cups water
1 cup tomatoes, diced
1 tsp. garlic, minced

Directions:
In a large pan over medium heat, add the olive oil, then brown the beef once it's hot.
Add the onion, tomatoes, garlic, cabbage, water, and broth.
Mix ingredients and bring to a boil. Add salt, pepper, and cumin powder.
Reduce the heat and let it simmer for 30 minutes.

Salmon Patties

(5 servings total; dinner)
(Per serving: 428 calories, 27 grams of fat, 48 grams of carbs, 38 grams of protein)

Ingredients:
2 eggs
Salt and pepper to taste
½ cup almond flour
2 tbsps. olive oil
1 tsp. lemon zest
4 oz. pork rinds, crushed
¼ cup grated Parmesan cheese
4 tbsps. dried herbs
2 cans pink salmon (~14.75 oz.)

Directions:
Drain both cans of the salmon and add to a mixing bowl.
Mix with the dried herbs, cheese, pork rinds, eggs, salt and pepper, and lemon zest.
Form into 10 evenly-sized balls.
Roll each ball in the almond flour until well coated.
Add olive oil to a skillet on medium heat.
Fry the patties for a few minutes on each side until golden brown.

Mustard Glazed Chicken Thighs

(3 servings total; dinner)
(Per serving: 190 calories, 12 grams of fat, 23 grams of protein, .8 grams of carbs)

Ingredients:
6 boneless chicken thighs
2 tbsps. coconut oil, melted
¾ tsp. poultry seasoning
Salt and pepper to taste
2 tbsps. low-carb mustard
Directions:
Preheat your oven to 425°F.
In a bowl, combine together the coconut oil, mustard, salt and pepper, and poultry seasoning.
Arrange the chicken into a baking sheet lined with parchment paper.
Brush the mustard glaze on top of each thigh and add extra seasoning if necessary.
Bake uncovered for 30 minutes.

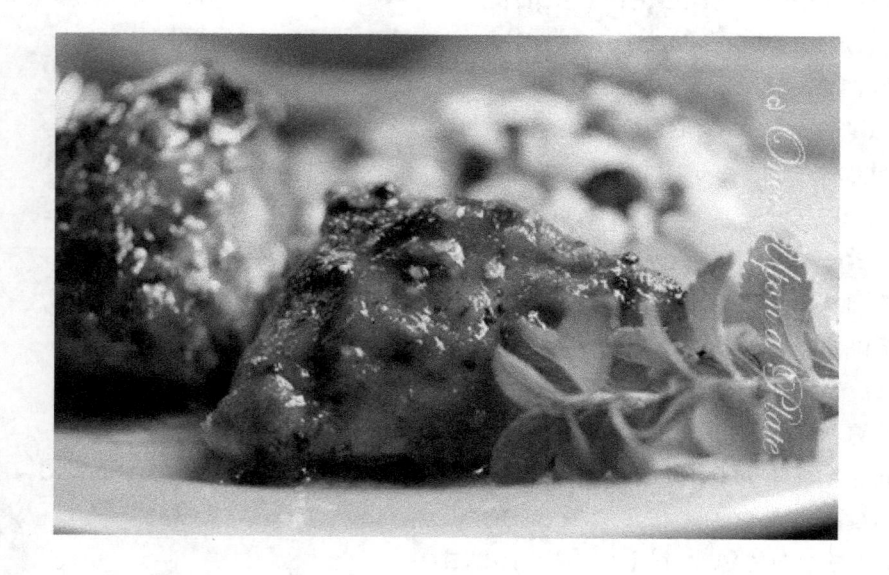

Romaine Lettuce Soup

(4 servings total; dinner)
(Per serving: 74 calories, 6 grams of fat, 4 grams of carbs, 1 gram of fiber, 1 gram of fiber)

Ingredients:
1 cup cauliflower, chopped
4 cups romaine lettuce, chopped
1 tbsp. ghee
2–3 garlic cloves, minced
½ cup onion, chopped
1 basil leaf, chopped
2 tbsps. fresh parsley, chopped
Salt and pepper to taste
2 cups chicken broth1.
Directions:
In a large saucepan on medium heat, add the ghee and sauté the onions and garlic.
Once the garlic is fragrant, add the basil and parsley, and season with salt and pepper.
Add the cauliflower, lettuce, and broth, and allow everything to simmer for about 15 minutes.
Use an immersion blender or a regular blender to puree everything into a smooth.
Add additional seasoning if necessary.
Low-Carb Chili (5 servings total; dinner)
(Per serving: 297 calories, 18 grams of fat, 24 grams of protein, 14 grams of carbs, 3 grams of fiber)
Ingredients:
1-pound ground beef

½ cup onion, chopped
3–4 garlic cloves, minced
1 tbsp. olive oil
1 can diced tomatoes (~15 oz.)
1 tbsp. Worcestershire sauce
3 tbsps. chili powder
1 tablespoon cumin powder
1 tbsp. dried herbs
Salt and pepper to taste

Directions:

In a large skillet over medium heat, add the olive oil and cook the onions until caramelized.
Add the garlic and cook until it's fragrant.
Add the ground beef and cook until it is brown.
Transfer the mixture to a crockpot or slow cooker.
Add the rest of the ingredients and stir until everything is well-combined.
Add salt and pepper to your taste. Cook for 5–6 hours on low or 3–4 hours on high.

Taco Salad Bowl

(3 servings total; dinner)
(Per serving: 178 calories, 12.8 grams of fat, 10 grams of protein, 2 grams of fiber, 4.8 grams of carbs)
Ingredients:
½ pound ground beef
1tbsp. avocado oil

1 tbsp. taco seasoning
4 oz. romaine lettuce, chopped
6–8 cherry tomatoes, sliced
¼ cup grated cheddar cheese
½ avocado, pitted, peeled, diced
3 tbsps. low-carb salsa
3 tbsps. sour cream
Salt and pepper to taste
Directions:
In a skillet on medium heat, add the avocado oil.
Add the ground beef and fry until it's golden brown.
Add in the taco seasoning and extra salt and pepper to taste.
Add to a bowl and mix with the remaining vegetables.
Top with salsa and sour cream.

Cauliflower Mac and Cheese

(4 servings total; dinner)
(Per serving: 324 calories, 32 grams of fat, 8 grams of carbs, 18 grams of protein)

Ingredients:
1 pound cauliflower florets
2 tbsps. olive oil
Salt and pepper to taste
¼ cup grated parmesan cheese
½ cup heavy cream
3 oz. grated cheddar cheese
2 oz. full-fat cream cheese
2 tsp. mustard
½ tsp. garlic powder
½ tsp. chili powder

Directions:
Preheat the oven to 400°F.
Make sure your cauliflower is in small bite-size pieces.
Spread out onto a baking sheet and drizzle with olive oil.
Bake for 15–20 minutes until the cauliflower becomes soft.
While the tray is in the oven, prepare the sauce in a small saucepan.
Add the last 7 ingredients to the saucepan and whisk until melted and smooth.
Keep the sauce warm while the cauliflower bakes.

In a large bowl, mix together the baked cauliflower and the cheese sauce.

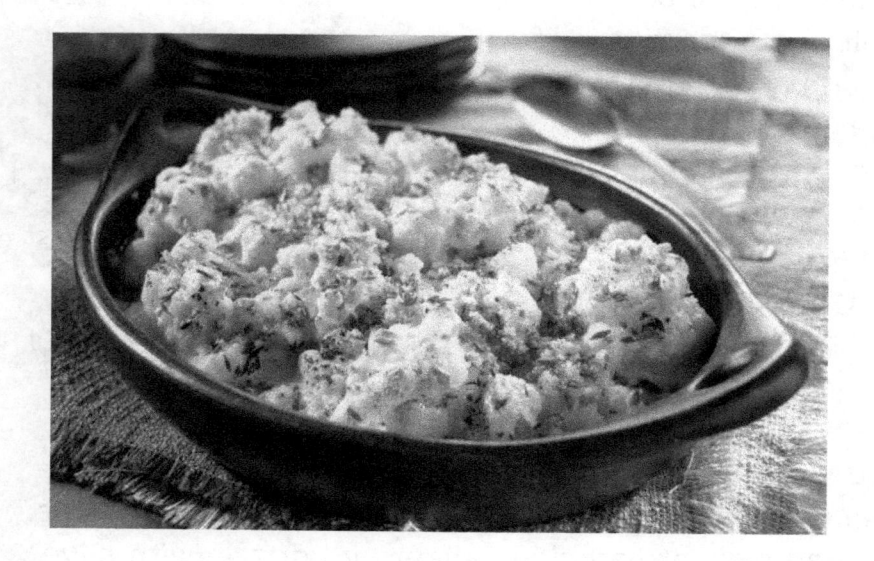

CPSIA information can be obtained
at www.ICGtesting.com
Printed in the USA
LVHW051711070221
678648LV00019B/767

9 781801 674331